Managing the
Patient-Centered Pharmacy

Managing the
Patient-Centered Pharmacy

Harry P. Hagel & John P. Rovers, Editors

American Pharmaceutical Association
Washington, D.C.

Acquiring Editor: Julian I. Graubart
Production Editor: Vicki Meade, Meade Communications
Assistant Editor: Mary De Angelo, Inkwell Communications
Layout and Graphics: Michele Danoff, Graphics by Design
Cover Design: Jim McDonald
Proofreader: Amy Morgante
Indexing: Suzanne Peake

To comment on this book via e-mail, send your message to the publisher at
aphabooks@mail.aphanet.org

Library of Congress Cataloging-in-Publication Data

Managing the patient-centered pharmacy / Harry P. Hagel and John P. Rovers, editors.
    p. ; cm.
  Includes bibliographical references and index.
  ISBN 1-58212-010-2
    1. Pharmacy management. I. Hagel, Harry P. II. Rovers, John P.
  [DNLM: 1. Pharmacy Administration. 2. Patient-Centered Care. QV 737 M2659 2002]
RS100 .M364 2002

2002018278

How to Order This Book
Online: www.pharmacist.com
By phone: 800-878-0729 (from the United States and Canada)
VISA®, MasterCard®, and American Express® cards accepted.

Dedication

This book is dedicated to the many pharmacists around the world who have shown us all that pharmacists are willing, capable, and successful at providing genuine care for their patients. These pioneers have been ingenious in finding ways around, over, under, or through the barriers that make the transition to patient-centered care difficult. They are an inspiration to pharmacists everywhere!

Contents

Foreword

An eclectic group of authors, including a couple of Aussies, gathered together and pooled their knowledge to produce this book. All 10 chapters are chock-full of detailed information on everything you ever wanted to know about providing enhanced patient care services, but were afraid to ask!

The authors apply strategic planning and business concepts to the process of developing professional patient care services. Throughout the book, they dissect the steps involved in implementing patient care, following a process-oriented approach as they explore the book's key themes. In several chapters, case examples give readers additional understanding of strategies for developing patient care services in various practice sites.

Chapter 3, on interdisciplinary patient care (IPC), was of particular interest to me because it details the "who, what, when, where, why, how, and how much" of starting up a patient care program. Wisely, the chapter notes that successful practitioners intuitively recognize that pharmaceutical care is not practiced in a vacuum. Instead, it is a cooperative partnership between the pharmacist, physician, and patient. A road map for developing a successful IPC partnership is well laid out, presenting all essential components from getting started to dealing with the challenges of reimbursement. The chapter emphasizes that positive relationships with other health care providers allow pharmacists to become essential members of the health care team.

Training, education, and motivation of pharmacists are necessary components of establishing and maintaining patient care services. *Managing the Patient-Centered Pharmacy* gives expert advice in these areas and offers examples of existing programs. The concepts of financial management, managing patient outcomes, and continuous quality improvement are each examined in separate chapters.

All pharmacists could benefit from reading this compendium of advice, strategies, and resources. Naturally, no one has every answer to the myriad questions that we, as professionals, encounter daily. Each author's personal expertise, however, and the blending of minds that produced this book give readers important insights into a "systemswide" approach to providing patient care services in today's pharmacy practice.

Dennis J. McCallian, PharmD
Professor, Community Pharmacy Practice
Director, Community Practice Development
Midwestern University College of Pharmacy
Glendale, Arizona

Contributors

Daniel H. Albrant, PharmD
Pharmacy Dynamics
Arlington, Virginia

Jana M. Bajcar, MS
Associate Professor of Pharmacy and
Director, Doctor of Pharmacy Program
University of Toronto
Toronto, Ontario, Canada

John M. Chapman, BPharm, BComm
National Director, Australian Institute
  of Pharmacy Management
Canberra, ACT, Australia

Karen B. Farris, PhD
Associate Professor of Pharmacy
University of Iowa
Iowa City, Iowa

Harry P. Hagel, MS
Integrated Pharmacy Strategies
Orlando, Florida

Ross W. Holland, PhD
Dean, Australian College of Pharmacy
  Practice
Canberra, ACT, Australia

June Felice Johnson, PharmD
Associate Professor and Vice-Chair
Department of Pharmacy Practice
Drake University
Des Moines, Iowa

Kathleen A. Johnson, PharmD, PhD
Associate Professor of Pharmacy
University of Southern California
Los Angeles, California

Lon N. Larson, PhD
Professor of Pharmacy Administration
Drake University
Des Moines, Iowa

Richard K. Lewis, PharmD, MBA
Mercy Resource Management Inc.
Naperville, Illinois

Christine M. Nimmo, PhD
Director, Educational Resources
American Society of Health-System
  Pharmacists
Bethesda, Maryland

Charles R. Phillips, PhD
Associate Professor of Pharmacy
  Administration
Drake University
Des Moines, Iowa

John P. Rovers, PharmD
Associate Professor of Pharmacy
Drake University
Des Moines, Iowa

Susan J. Skledar, MPH
Assistant Director, Drug Use and
  Disease State Management Program
University of Pittsburgh Medical
  Center Health System
Pittsburgh, Pennsylvania

Introduction

Harry P. Hagel & John P. Rovers

Why is it that, even though pharmacists say they want to provide patient care, few actually do it? In the decade since the pharmaceutical care philosophy was introduced, countless pharmacists have expressed interest in changing their practices to focus on patient care. But despite the many resources on hand to help, change has been slow and difficult.

Ultimately, both pharmacists *and* systems need to change. Workshops, books, videos, and software help pharmacists improve their knowledge and skills, but what about creating an environment that supports patient care? We wrote this book to enable owners, managers, and pharmacy executives to change the systems within pharmacies so a patient-focused practice can emerge.

From Distribution to Patient Care

For most of pharmacy's history, the pharmacist's role was to procure, store, prepare, and provide drug products for treating patients' illnesses. By the 1950s, however, the drug manufacturing industry had largely taken over the first three responsibilities and pharmacists were left to focus on the last one—providing drug products to patients.

Pharmacists have always spent a lot of time talking with patients about their medicines and answering questions, but since the middle of the last century most of our job and virtually all of our income has depended on supplying drug products to people who need them. A fairly small number of pharmacists practiced what was called "clinical pharmacy," most often in an inpatient setting, but clinical pharmacy services were rarely available to patients everywhere. Instead, most pharmacists, regardless of where we worked, were usually behind the prescription counter preparing medications for patients.

Pharmacy was reasonably successful in this practice mode until the 1980s, when rapidly escalating health care costs gave rise to managed care. Suddenly, the marketplace was only interested in buying pills as cheaply as possible. The old model of making money by selling drugs for more than we paid for them was thrown out the window. Payers no longer asked, "What does it cost?" Instead, they told us, "Here's what we'll pay."

Introduction

At about the same time, a fast-growing body of evidence began to show that using medications improperly is expensive—and not just in dollars. We learned that medication problems are more prevalent than we'd recognized, and they can result in illness, lost productivity, and death. Furthermore, we realized that no one in health care has specific responsibility for ensuring that medications do what they are supposed to do.

In the early 1990s, pharmacy visionaries proposed a new practice approach in which pharmacists would get paid for ensuring that drugs bring about positive results. This patient-centered model of practice is called pharmaceutical care.

Unfortunately, changing from a product-focused business to a patient-centered practice model is much harder than we first envisioned. Thousands of pharmacists have successfully transformed their practices to provide patient services ranging from self-care advising to disease management clinics. But thousands more continue to battle on the front lines with larger-than-ever prescription volumes, declining reimbursement levels, and staff shortages. Although many struggling pharmacists try to enhance their patient care skills, the system they work in is not conducive to the changes they want to bring about.

Why We Wrote This Book

We developed this book to help owners, managers, executives, and pharmacy staffs gear up for pharmaceutical care. In these pages you learn how to refocus systems—from developing a new practice vision to adjusting infrastructure and managing your finances. This book takes a global view, addressing pharmacists in all settings. It targets change at the practice rather than the individual level.

Readers not yet familiar with the practice functions necessary to provide pharmaceutical care should do some background study before applying the principles in this book. Our previous book, *A Practical Guide to Pharmaceutical Care* (Washington, D.C.: American Pharmaceutical Association; 1998), written with colleagues from the Iowa Center for Pharmaceutical Care—Jay Currie, Randy McDonough, and Jenelle Sobotka—presents clear principles, methods, and examples for providing pharmaceutical care.

How to Use This Book

Each chapter discusses the most important management topics for implementing or improving patient services. The material helps you think through problems associated with various changes and offers guidance for creating a practice change plan.

It's best to read the entire book first to become familiar with patient-centered pharmacy management principles and identify specific issues in your practice. Then you can return to individual chapters to study and apply them. Taking notes in the page margins, highlighting key portions of text, or creating lists of strategies you find especially relevant may help you make the most of the book.

Four Key Questions

This book is organized to help you answer four primary questions. "Where am I now?" focuses on the operational capacity of your practice to address the pharmaceutical care needs of patients. Once you know where you are, you should be able to give an honest and thorough answer to the second question, "Where do I want to be?" Achieving meaningful, lasting change in your practice will be difficult without knowing where you are going and what goal you want to reach. Responding to the third question, "How do I get there?" requires that you apply the management principles discussed in various chapters. To answer the final question, "How will I know when I have reached my destination?" you must integrate patient outcomes, financial data, and quality improvement systems into your patient service programs. The table below identifies chapters that are most useful for answering each strategic planning question.

Guide to Answering Strategic Planning Questions	
Where am I now?	Chapter 1: Planning for Patient Care
Where do I want to be?	Chapter 2: Changing Your Practice for Patient Care
How do I get there?	Chapter 3: Interdisciplinary Patient Care
	Chapter 4: Developing the Infrastructure for Patient Care
	Chapter 5: Motivating Staff for Patient Care
	Chapter 6: Education and Training for Patient Care
	Chapter 7: Creating a Business Plan for Patient Care
How will I know when I have reached my destination?	Chapter 8: Financial Management for Patient Care
	Chapter 9: Managing Patient Outcome Data
	Chapter 10: Continuous Quality Improvement

Who Should Read This Book

Anyone responsible for implementing patient services, maximizing or justifying pharmacy resources, or demonstrating the value of pharmacy services can benefit from this book. If you are a pharmacist, a pharmacy owner, a student soon entering practice, a pharmacy manager in a hospital or community setting, or a health care executive responsible for pharmacy operations, you will find this book immediately relevant. The book's insights also apply to pharmacists working in a managed care environment, long-term care pharmacy, specialty compounding pharmacy, or college of pharmacy.

Hospital Pharmacy Directors and Managers

Trying to do more with less is the reality today. Faced with competing priorities, pharmacy directors and managers may find it extremely difficult to put new or expanded services in place. However, capitated hospital payment contracts, rising medication costs, and increasingly severe drug therapy problems only reinforce the need for you to use resources judiciously. This book can help you:

+ Develop an action plan to contain costs.
+ Learn how to establish a quality improvement program.
+ Create interdisciplinary teams.
+ Improve staff recruitment, development, and retention.
+ Justify new automation and technology.
+ Document the financial and clinical impact of new services.

Community Pharmacy Owners, Managers, and Executives

With third-party reimbursement shrinking, more providers competing for health care dollars, and new drug-distribution models emerging, community pharmacies must explore ways to differentiate themselves in the marketplace. This book helps you:

+ Evaluate your customers' needs.
+ Determine the type of services to offer.
+ Develop a business plan.
+ Establish financial systems to obtain capital funding.
+ Track financial performance.
+ Evaluate the impact of care.

Employee Pharmacists

Given the day-to-day volatility of both health care and the pharmacy profession, one prediction sure to hold true is that things will keep changing. If you possess the skills and tenacity to change, you are more likely to enjoy a productive, rewarding career. Delivering high-quality patient services and understanding the associated management issues will bring you more opportunities for growth and leadership. This book offers concrete information to shape your professional destiny.

Health Care Executives and Administrators

Pharmaceutical budgets represent a growing percentage of total health care costs. Controlling these budgets is a concern shared by everyone in health care management, from managed care organizations to national, regional, and local health systems. This book gives tips for using pharmacists more effectively to manage costs related to unsafe and ineffective medication use. It also helps you identify resources and organizational support within your pharmacy operations to save money while improving the quality of patient care.

Pharmacy Faculty and Students

As the demand for patient services expands, the pharmacy profession needs energetic, knowledgeable new practitioners willing to accept the challenges of change. You can integrate material from this book into pharmacy curricula and use it as a discussion tool at experiential teaching sites.

A Final Thought

It has been our distinct honor to edit this book and to work with the exceptionally talented authors who contributed their knowledge, expertise, and insight. We believe you will find this information usable, understandable, and relevant for the practice of pharmacy today and for several years ahead. Anyone who buys this book probably has a vision for practice that reaches firmly into the realm of patient care. We share that vision, and we wish you a long and productive journey towards a rewarding patient-centered pharmacy practice.

Chapter 1
PLANNING FOR PATIENT CARE
Harry P. Hagel

If you are reading this book, you probably have a nagging awareness that you should be providing enhanced patient care services within your pharmacy. Or perhaps you're responding to a management directive. Regardless of the reason, you have to apply a strategic planning process—which has been taught in business schools for decades—to fundamentally change your pharmacy's practice model. This chapter will not present a detailed theoretical discussion of strategic planning, a topic covered in countless textbooks. Instead, it will help you incorporate the information presented in subsequent chapters into a comprehensive plan for creating, implementing, and improving patient services. If you take the time to answer four basic questions, you will be well on your way to creating a detailed road map. These questions are: Where are you now? Where do you want to be? How will you reach your destination? How will you know when you have arrived?

Where Are You Now?

When formulating a plan for patient care, you should start by determining the present level of services you provide. You also need to identify the internal and external factors that affect your efforts—or that have the potential to affect them. In strategic planning jargon this activity is often referred to as a "SWOT" analysis, which looks at strengths, weaknesses, opportunities, and threats. To develop patient care services, you should concentrate your SWOT analysis on major practice elements that pharmacists employ in providing patient care. Doing this requires you to obtain sufficient input from the people directly and indirectly affected by the new services.

To assess your current practice, start by identifying the strengths, weakness, opportunities, and threats related to each element in the box on page 2. These elements are explored thoroughly in Form 1-1, the Practice Assessment SWOT Analysis Worksheet at the end of this chapter. Complete Form 1-1 after you have carefully read Chapter 2 of this book. The SWOT worksheet will guide you through a structured review of your current practice environment and marketplace so that you can later identify strategies for achieving your patient care vision.

To improve the usefulness and accuracy of your practice assessment, solicit input from anyone currently involved in your practice and anyone you intend to collaborate with in providing patient care. In some instances you may find it helpful to conduct surveys, work-sampling studies, and personal interviews. Regardless of your methods, the most important factor when completing a practice assessment is to obtain honest feedback from customers, colleagues, friends, and other professional contacts relevant to your core business.

Completing Your Practice Assessment

As indicated in the SWOT analysis sidebar below, practice assessment can be divided into two major areas. Internal practice elements include current pharmacy services, operations, and human resource issues that reflect your current ability and eventual capacity to provide individualized patient care. The second area focuses on patient characteristics, relationships with prescribers or other providers, and the payer environment for patient care services. Let's begin by examining the internal practice elements.

Internal Capacity Factors: Strengths and Weaknesses

Pharmacy Services

By conducting a thorough inventory of the types and quality of services currently provided by your pharmacy, you can determine the foundation on which to build future services. When evaluating existing services, consider whether they are patient- or product-focused, whether they are provided reliably and consistently, and how they are perceived by people who receive or purchase them. If you already have effective, high-quality services, a reasonable next step is to add or expand your services. However, if you determine that an existing service is substandard in quality or provided inconsistently to patients, you should first focus on improving what you have rather than developing new services.

SWOT Analysis Elements

Internal Capacity Factors
(strengths and weaknesses)
+ Pharmacy services
+ Pharmacy operations
+ Human resources

External Demand Factors
(opportunities and threats)
+ Patient characteristics
+ Prescriber/provider relations
+ Payer environment

Pharmacy Operations

Pharmacists most commonly cite lack of time as their biggest barrier to providing additional patient services. Because today's practices are so busy, most pharmacies will need to re-engineer their workflow and staffing methods to free pharmacists' time for patient interaction. To accomplish this, you must first determine how effectively your pharmacy uses technicians and other support personnel to perform tasks that do not require a pharmacist's education and training. Second, you should look at the extent to which your pharmacy integrates automation and technology into its distributive and clinical functions. Third, you should consider whether your pharmacy's physical environment is conducive to interacting effectively with patients. And last, you must assess the pharmacy's financial resources, data management systems, business plans, and policies and procedures to determine how well they can support new patient services.

Human Resources

Oftentimes, patient care ventures are limited by the availability of motivated, competent pharmacists and technicians who accept the challenge of providing patient care services. Therefore, you must carefully evaluate your current human resources. Assess the staff's competence, communication skills, motivation, and professionalism. Determine how well the pharmacists and technicians work together as a team, and examine the effectiveness of your retention and recruitment efforts.

External Demand Factors: Opportunities and Threats
Patient Characteristics

Although it may be possible for you to generate demand for a totally new service, you probably will find it more efficient to first determine the current needs of existing customers and build from there. Begin by evaluating your prescription or hospital census data to estimate the number of patients with various medical conditions. Consider whether their prescribed therapy is consistent with current treatment guidelines. What types of drug therapy problems does each patient group experience? What questions and concerns do patients tend to bring up? What ages, gender, and socioeconomic groups typically seek advice from the pharmacist? What are the health beliefs and health care purchasing patterns for these patient groups? Understanding your patients' concerns, beliefs, and wants will reduce your risk of developing services that are either unnecessary or not desired by your customer base.

Prescriber and Provider Relations

Because licensed physicians or other authorized providers must prescribe the prescription drugs that your patients receive, it seems logical to closely examine your relationships with these professionals. Not only are patients usually more willing to cooperate with new services that are backed by their doctors, but you are more likely to get reimbursed by insurance companies when physicians can certify the medical necessity of your services. You can also bring about greater benefits for patients with similar drug therapy needs and problems by coordinating care with other providers.

Think about this: do prescribers and other health care providers seek out the pharmacists in your organization for drug information, advice, or assistance with problem patients? If so, building upon existing relationships and developing new ones can become a valuable source of patient referrals and continual business growth.

Payer Environment

From the start, you must consider how you will sustain the new service venture financially. Even in hospital environments with capitated payment structures, you must look beyond cost savings to ways you can generate a revenue stream. Consider patients your number one prospect for revenue. After all, they are the ultimate recipients of the new service, and unless *they* perceive it to be of value—which they demonstrate by paying for it—it is unlikely that the medical payer community will eventually agree to large-scale reimbursement.

In recent years, the reimbursement climate has been changing for pharmacists. Large employers, third-party payers, and even physician groups at risk for excess health care expenditures are beginning to pay pharmacists for a variety of services. Rising health care costs and skyrocketing prescription prices are forcing many payers to examine methods for improving utilization and outcomes of drug therapy. This trend represents a golden revenue-producing opportunity for pharmacy practices.

Pharmaceutical manufacturers, who frequently support specific projects such as disease screening and management programs, offer another potential source of revenue. Medical and pharmacy researchers need pharmacy providers to evaluate new therapies or service delivery models and often provide modest payment. In addition, state and national practice associations sometimes pay pharmacists who participate in regional or national demonstration projects. Be creative when identifying potential payers who may fit well into your professional and business network.

Where Do You Want to Be?

Most pharmacists agree that the pharmacy profession's purpose in society includes caring for the medication-related needs of patients. Pharmacy and medical literature contains many examples of pharmacists providing exemplary patient care, and pharmacists' achievements are proudly described at professional pharmacy meetings in the United States and abroad. So why do consumers, prescribers, and other health care providers hesitate to recognize pharmacists' tremendous potential for enhancing patient care?

Instead of examining the many reasons why pharmacy is struggling to solidify its patient care role, let's focus on a key solution: ensuring that pharmacists' compassion, genuine concern for patients' well-being, and desire to help people achieve better health is consistently embraced and communicated within individual practices. When pharmacy staff change their attitudes and behaviors and begin to embrace a new patient care paradigm, patients notice the services they provide and start asking for them. You can lay the groundwork for these changes by creating a vision and a mission for patient care, as described in the following pages. By demonstrating to patients the actual care you provide, you can help overcome their hesitations about pharmacists' expanded role in the health care system.

Creating a Mission and Vision for Patient Care
Step 1: Identify Patient Service Goals

Once you identify both your personal and professional patient care goals, you can actually begin to convert your dreams into reality. Start by asking yourself a difficult question: "Why should I or the pharmacy I am responsible for provide a greater level of patient care than we offer now?" There are no right or wrong answers to this question. Your responses may include wanting to address community health needs, help individual patients achieve better health, improve customer loyalty and satisfaction, or simply generate additional revenue. Typically you will have multiple goals, but be careful not to begin with too many. Also, make sure you state your goals in a way that lets you measure the results. Having too many goals can lead to frustration, and you may become discouraged if you can't measure your progress within a reasonable time frame.

If you are responsible for managing pharmacist and technician staff in your pharmacy, it will also be important to identify their respective goals. Understanding individual staff goals and helping them recognize ways they can meet their goals by providing patient care will help you gain the support you need to develop and implement new services.

To identify your patient service goals, find some quiet, uninterrupted time—perhaps while you are driving to work—or specifically set aside time during your day to reflect on what you want. Keep in mind that goals are nothing more than the words you choose to describe what you want the practice to become. And don't limit the number and variety of goals you come up with. For example, goals for your pharmacy practice can include:

- Developing a smoking cessation program.
- Providing care to 25 patients in the first year of service.
- Receiving four referrals a month from local physicians who send patients to your pharmacotherapy evaluation clinic.

To identify goals for an entire pharmacy operation, you can begin with informal staff discussions and follow up with a scheduled meeting time to complete the goal-setting process. In some cases, a confidential staff survey can help elicit goals from individual staff members. Whatever means you use to pinpoint both your individual and organizational goals, write them down. This gives you clarity and helps you measure success later as you implement your plan for new patient care services. Share

Steps in Creating a Patient Care Mission and Vision

Step 1: Identify patient service goals. Do not begin with too many, and state them in measurable ways. Seek honest, objective feedback on your goals.

Step 2: Envision a patient care practice. Think about what you want to achieve. This is similar to imagining your destination when you embark on a journey, and deciding what you want to do when you get there.

Step 3: Write a patient service mission statement. This statement should answer the question, "What business are you in?" or "What is the overall reason your organization exists?"

Step 4: Communicate your mission to stakeholders. Let employees, customers, prescribers, payers, suppliers, stockholders, and others know what they can expect from you and your organization.

Step 5: Use your mission to make decisions. The mission provides a framework for deciding whether potential actions are right for your organization.

your goals with a friend, spouse, colleague, or business partner to obtain objective and honest feedback.

Step 2: Envision a Patient Care Practice

A "vision" can be described as what you eventually want to create or achieve. Once you have established your patient service goals, describe the practice environment, operational elements, and professional culture that will help you achieve each goal. This process is similar to selecting a trip destination, defining the purpose of the trip, and deciding what you want to do when you get there.

For example, your vision may be to implement automated and technician-driven drug distribution processes that enable pharmacists to spend most of their time helping patients and other health care providers achieve the best results from medication use. Begin by imagining what your practice must look like to accomplish your goals. If you are responsible for multiple pharmacy staff, engage them in a group exercise to identify specific practice attributes that will allow the practice to meet individual and collective goals. A shared vision is absolutely essential for an organization to move toward that vision.

Take time to imagine the ideal professional work environment for the practice you envision, including:

- The types of pharmacist-patient interactions that will take place.
- How technicians will support the drug distribution and patient care processes.

- Specific kinds of patient services you want to offer.
- Desired relationships with prescribers, other providers, and employers in your community.
- Forms of professional recognition you would find gratifying.

Remember, your vision should reflect your goals, such as providing care to a certain number of patients per month. You may also want to include additional practice elements and functions in your vision, such as implementing an automated dispensing system to free pharmacists' time for patient care. Approach the vision process with creativity and enthusiasm, while making every attempt to disregard barriers to reaching your goals.

Step 3: Write a Patient Service Mission Statement

In contrast to an organizational vision—which can be likened to a destination—a mission is the driving force behind the actions necessary to achieve the vision. A mission is not the specific actions you need to undertake, however. Instead, the mission answers the question "What business are you in?" or "What is the overall reason your organization exists?" If you already have a personal mission statement, or if your pharmacy already has one, evaluate whether each one truly reflects a patient care philosophy. When you evaluate an existing mission statement or develop a new one for an organization, it's important to get input from each staff member who will be expected to carry out the mission.

A well-developed mission statement will not only give direction and purpose to your professional practice, but it will also communicate what customers and stakeholders can expect from you. Include several of the following elements when writing your patient service mission statement:

- **Intended customers.** Who do you intend to offer your services to? In most instances, your primary customers will be the patients you interact with daily in your practice. But your customers may also include stakeholders that will benefit from or be affected by your mission, such as prescribers, other providers, payers, and employers.
- **Core values.** Core values reflect how you intend to deal with customers or how you will act when working towards your vision. Consider the values you desire in dealing with other health care providers such as compassion, respect, honesty, and confidentiality.
- **Services and products.** Concisely describe the general nature of the services you will offer. Use tangible descriptions, such as education or counseling sessions, health screening, or assistance with medication use. Avoid general terms such as "pharmacist patient care" or "pharmaceutical care," which mean nothing to nonpharmacists.

- **Goals and philosophies.** Develop a statement about the customer-related benefits that the patient services will achieve. State the service goals in a way that communicates specific benefits to the customer, such as better health, reduced costs, improved safety, or maximum effectiveness from proper medication use.
- **Desired public image.** Make sure the patient care mission conveys how you want to be viewed by the public and reinforces a primary focus on patient needs rather than on product sales or business success.

The sidebar below gives examples of patient service mission statements for a community and a hospital pharmacy. Both statements clearly communicate that the patient is the intended customer. Although the statements represent different practice settings, both convey a primary goal of safe and effective medication use. The community mission reinforces the professionalism of the staff, while the hospital mission reinforces the goal of coordinated care during and after the hospital stay. A patient, prescriber, or payer can readily determine what to expect from either pharmacy.

Sample Mission Statements

Representative Community Pharmacy is dedicated to helping patients achieve better health through safe and effective medication use. Our pharmacists and technicians are highly trained, compassionate professionals who provide comprehensive patient counseling and education services.

Representative Hospital Pharmacy is dedicated to achieving the best possible medication-related outcomes for our patients. Our primary aim is to ensure the availability and optimal use of drugs during a patient's stay in the hospital and the coordination of their drug therapy needs after discharge.

Step 4: Communicate Your Mission to Stakeholders

A stakeholder is any person or organization that is impacted by what you or your organization does. Potential stakeholders include employees, customers, prescribers, payers, the marketplace, suppliers, and in some cases, stockholders. Some stakeholders may already be involved in creating the vision and writing the mission statement, but others may not yet be aware of what you are trying to achieve (the vision) or how you intend to conduct yourself (the mission). Therefore, it is important to share your mission statement with others. This process is not self-promotion. Rather, sharing your mission makes you accountable and tells current and prospective stakeholders what they can expect from you or your organization. As a result, stakeholders can better understand the personal and business benefits of associating with your organization. Also, sharing your mission allows stakeholders to contribute new ideas to your vision and promotes a sense of commonality.

You can use a variety of media formats and methods to communicate your mission. Everyone in your organization should be able to verbally recite and describe the mission. Include your mission statement on marketing materials and display it on signage for customers and employees alike. Consider devoting some of your advertising dollars to promoting your new mission. Create bag stuffers that describe the mission and make sure that all customers receive one. Have staff wear "Ask me about our new mission" buttons to prompt patients to inquire about what you're doing. Be creative and patient. It can be hard to get people's attention, given all the marketing messages they are exposed to daily. Remember, your goal is to make patients notice you are improving your practice.

Step 5: Use Your Mission to Make Decisions
The final—and probably most important—aspect of creating a patient care mission is to keep the mission alive and use it to guide your practice management decisions. Once you have a mission statement in place, use it to answer questions such as: Is your decision to send a pharmacist or technician to a professional meeting, purchase new inventory, or hire a particular staff person consistent with the mission? Will a new business venture you are considering enhance your mission?

A well defined mission gives you and your staff clarity when making operational and patient care decisions each day. The mission serves as a frame of reference when you evaluate long-range planning considerations such as resource allocation, new service development, employee performance, staff recruitment, and marketing initiatives.

Taking the time to create a vision and mission for patient care is a critical step to reaching your full potential as a health care provider. Although most pharmacists already have a subconscious vision and carry out their daily practice responsibilities with commendable professionalism and duty, completing the steps described above can enhance your sense of purpose and provide direction for future endeavors.

Defining Your Patient Service
Defining what patient services are most appropriate for your specific practice can be confusing. Pharmacy literature uses many different terms to describe the patient care services provided by pharmacists, such as disease management, pharmacist care, and cognitive services. Additionally, the American Pharmaceutical Association describes the process of pharmacist patient care as:

℞ Service Development Questions

+ What type of patients need additional services from your pharmacists?

+ What drug therapy problems commonly affect the target patient population?

+ What is the best way to prevent or resolve the drug therapy problems typically encountered in the target patient group?

+ What specific patient information will your pharmacists need to uncover potential or existing drug therapy problems in the target patient group?

+ To effectively provide care to patients, what skills will your pharmacists need?

+ What forms and patient record systems will you need?

+ What written material or other resources will you provide to the patient?

+ What are the best methods and where is the best location for your pharmacists to interact with patients?

+ Will you schedule patient meetings with the pharmacist on specific days or at specific times?

continued on page 11

1. Collecting patient-specific data.
2. Evaluating data to identify drug therapy problems.
3. Developing a plan to correct or prevent drug therapy problems.
4. Implementing a plan of care.
5. Monitoring the care plan for desired patient outcomes.

Although this definition of care is widely accepted, it helps to translate the steps into an actual, tangible process. Begin by answering the service development questions in the sidebar to the left as completely as possible. Focus on how you would *ideally* provide the service. Do not worry about how you will *actually* put the service into practice or what barriers may exist, since formulating strategies for successful implementation is the next step in the planning process.

When you finish answering the service development questions, you should have a comprehensive description of the patients you intend to target, how you will provide your services, and how you will document and get reimbursed for care. Chapter 2 elaborates on this topic and presents a complete discussion of selecting and developing a patient service model.

How Will You Reach Your Destination?

Now that you know where you are and where you want to go, it's time to embark on your journey. In this phase, you will formulate and implement strategies to complete the tasks you identified in the service development exercise.

Service Development Questions, continued

✦ How and when will you handle patient monitoring and follow-up?

✦ How much time will you require for the initial patient consultation and for follow-up sessions?

✦ What legal and regulatory requirements exist for patient referrals, care protocols, documentation, and reimbursement?

✦ What methods will you use to document patient care activities so that you ensure continuity of care and demonstrate patient outcomes?

✦ How and when will you coordinate care or communicate with the patient's physician or other health care providers?

However, this is not just a matter of building a consultation area, installing a computerized documentation system, developing a patient brochure, or undertaking additional training.

As you decide exactly how to proceed, take into account the results of your SWOT analysis. Determine which practice elements already exist to support the new service and what else needs to be done. For example, if the intended target group is patients with diabetes, make sure that you have the necessary physical setup, monitoring equipment, documentation system, and clinical skills before you actually begin marketing your services to patients or other referral sources. Depending on the location of your practice, you will also need to initiate care protocols, collaborative practice agreements, and direct patient or third-party billing procedures.

For each task you need to complete, figure out the best approach. For example, billing third-party payers means that you may need a certificate of medical necessity for specific procedures or that you must have a formalized patient care protocol in place. If this is the case, you will need a comprehensive strategy for establishing open communication and ensuring support from prescribers. To set up the agreements you need, you may want to hold meetings with prescribers to discuss how you can work together to improve medication use for patients common to your practices. Building trust and relationships can take time and require a succession of meetings. As this example illustrates, any strategy you undertake for completing the tasks revealed by your SWOT analysis may require multiple steps and considerable time.

Developing a Work Plan

To avoid getting lost on your journey to patient care, track progress and identify potential detours by using an organized work plan. Create a table with at least 13 columns: one column for the task and the remaining columns for each of the next 12 months. Estimate how long you think it will take to complete each task, and fill in the associated number of months. Some tasks need to be completed before you can proceed to others, so you must prioritize each of your tasks as you complete the table. A completed work plan may look like the template in Figure 1-1.

Figure 1-1. Work Plan Template

Tasks and Strategies	Person Responsible	Est. Cost	Completion Date	Implementation Month											
				1	2	3	4	5	6	7	8	9	10	11	12
TASK 1				▒	▒	▒	▒	▒							
Strategy 1-1				▒	▒										
Strategy 1-2							▒	▒							
TASK 2										▒	▒	▒	▒	▒	▒
Strategy 2-1										▒	▒				
Strategy 2-2												▒	▒		
TASK 3													▒	▒	

After generating a timetable in your work plan, you must determine the cost of completing each individual task. Think about materials, personnel, time, travel costs, and perhaps even the present value of money if it affects other revenue-generating activity. If you are not completing all tasks yourself, identify who will be responsible, agree upon the completion date, and decide what evidence you will use to confirm completion. Finally, share your work plan with everyone involved to get feedback, support, advice, and encouragement. This will also force you to be accountable. If you don't tell anyone what you intend to do and when you plan to begin, it becomes easy to circumvent your work plan and focus instead on other day-to-day priorities. To help you and everyone else remain positive and committed to the plan, remember to celebrate completed milestones and reward both individual and group efforts.

How Will You Know When You Have Arrived?

It's now time to see if you have met your goals. If your goals are vague or if you don't have any, you'll have a hard time determining if you've successfully changed your practice. But if you have explicitly defined your service objectives in terms of both operations and patient outcomes, you will have measurable parameters for assessing your new patient services.

If your operational objectives are financial, for example, you could set up an accounting system for tracking income and expenses related to the new service. You could also look at the volume of documented pharmacist activities, number of patient referrals, or increases in prescription volume.

The goals you set for patient outcomes may fall into any of three areas: economic, clinical, and humanistic. Economic elements include changes in average prescription drug costs for the target patient group, reductions in medical expenditures, and less employee absenteeism. Clinical elements include laboratory or physical assessment markers of drug efficacy and safety. Typically, you measure humanistic outcomes using validated quality of life instruments that assess the physical and psychological factors that influence the patient's overall health and well-being. Chapters 8 and 9 offer advice on collecting and using financial and patient-related outcomes data.

If you use computer-based documentation systems, you will find that they make data collection and analysis much easier. You should record and track data about patient demographics, payers, prescribers, drug utilization, billing, productivity, drug therapy problems, health care utilization, specific diseases, and drug therapy outcomes. Analyzing this data can give you key information for improving the quality of your services, making practice management decisions, designing marketing campaigns, and getting reimbursed from third-party payers.

Next Steps

Although this chapter provides a helpful template to get you started, in each subsequent chapter experienced practitioners, managers, and researchers guide you through the process of creating a plan for patient care. Chapter 2 describes the steps involved in changing the focus and culture of your practice. Chapter 3 covers how to create interdisciplinary care teams. Chapter 4 looks at developing such operational elements as automation and technology, the physical environment, and policies and procedures. Chapters 5 and 6 give invaluable insights into human resource issues such as motivation and training. Chapters 7 and 8 present a concise, easy-to-understand approach to business planning, marketing, and financial systems that can help you obtain funding and track implementation success. Chapter 9 offers a detailed discussion about the collection, analysis, and reporting of patient outcome data, and Chapter 10 describes how to use data for continuous quality improvement.

Creating a plan for patient care requires motivation and effort. Your diligence, combined with this book's guidance, provide the basic ingredients for formulating a workable plan to launch new patient care services.

Form 1-1. Practice Assessment SWOT Analysis Worksheet

Instructions:

For each practice assessment element listed in the following worksheet, indicate whether it is a strength, weakness, opportunity or threat to your ability to provide individualized patient care services. Where applicable, make any relevant notes or comments. You may want to have others complete the worksheet as part of a group meeting. You could also adapt the content for survey instruments or use it as a guideline for conducting personal interviews with key business stakeholders.

INTERNAL CAPACITY FACTORS

PHARMACY SERVICES	ANALYSIS	COMMENTS/NOTES
Provide individual patient disease management consults but do not receive reimbursement.	S W O T	
Provide individual patient disease management consults and receive reimbursement.	S W O T	
Provide face-to-face patient counseling to patients receiving new prescriptions.	S W O T	
Provide face-to-face patient counseling to patients receiving refill prescriptions.	S W O T	
Offer prescription delivery services at no charge.	S W O T	
Offer prescription delivery services for a fee.	S W O T	
Provide consulting services to long-term care patients.	S W O T	
Offer group or individualized patient education programs on specific drug or disease topics.	S W O T	
Provide community education programs on health-related topics.	S W O T	
Assist and educate patients selecting nonprescription products and medical devices.	S W O T	
Pharmacist is always available to patients and prescribers for answering questions, dispensing emergency medications, or resolving drug therapy problems.	S W O T	
Maintain written documentation of services provided to patients, which can be retrieved, reviewed, and analyzed to assess impact on patient medication outcomes.	S W O T	

continued on page 15

INTERNAL CAPACITY FACTORS, continued

PHARMACY SERVICES	ANALYSIS	COMMENTS/NOTES
Conduct individual patient drug therapy reviews but do not receive reimbursement.	S W O T	
Conduct individual patient drug therapy reviews and receive reimbursement.	S W O T	
Provide specific clinical services for designated inpatients.	S W O T	
Pharmacist is involved in patient care at the point of prescribing by the physician.	S W O T	
Pharmacist is involved in developing medication formulary and clinical use guidelines.	S W O T	
Pharmacy participates in formalized education programs for students and/or residents.	S W O T	
Medication dispensing is accurate and consistent with professional standards and legal requirements.	S W O T	
Medication dispensing is efficient and consistent with professional standards and legal requirements.	S W O T	
Pharmacy services are consistent with professional guidelines on providing pharmaceutical care to patients.	S W O T	

INTERNAL CAPACITY FACTORS

PHARMACY OPERATIONS	ANALYSIS	COMMENTS/NOTES
Supervised pharmacy technicians perform the majority of dispensing-related tasks.	S W O T	
Supervised pharmacy technicians or clerks perform product inventory and office-related functions.	S W O T	
Pharmacy space is designed to maximize efficiency and reduce redundant or unnecessary staff work motions.	S W O T	
Automation and technology are integral components of both dispensing and clinical-related functions.	S W O T	
Policies and procedures are in place to ensure consistency and quality in operational tasks.	S W O T	

continued on page 16

INTERNAL CAPACITY FACTORS, continued

PHARMACY OPERATIONS	ANALYSIS	COMMENTS/NOTES
Prescription processing follows a designated workflow from start to finish.	S W O T	
Staffing levels are consistent with prescription volume and other pharmacy workload patterns.	S W O T	
The pharmacist workload allows for patients to ask questions or request assistance.	S W O T	
Drug information resources are up-to-date and easily accessible for review by pharmacy staff.	S W O T	
The pharmacy has designated areas for receiving prescription orders and for processing and dispensing medications.	S W O T	
A comfortable and separate waiting area for patients is located near the prescription dispensing area.	S W O T	
A private area for patient consultation is easily accessible by both pharmacists and patients and is close to other health-related products and information.	S W O T	
A pharmacist workspace separate from the dispensing area is available to make phone calls, review drug literature, and engage in professional development activities.	S W O T	
The pharmacy environment is clean and organized and reflects a health care image.	S W O T	
Financial management systems are in place to track the performance of specific services.	S W O T	
A comprehensive business plan for patient services has been developed.	S W O T	
Legal and regulatory standards are conducive to pharmacists providing patient care services.	S W O T	

continued on page 17

INTERNAL CAPACITY FACTORS

HUMAN RESOURCES	ANALYSIS	COMMENTS/NOTES
Pharmacists are competent to provide the specific patient care services under consideration for development/implementation.	S W O T	
Pharmacists are credentialed and/or certified in specific disease management areas or other specialized services.	S W O T	
Pharmacists understand their role in patient care and willingly accept responsibility for improving patients' medication-related health.	S W O T	
Pharmacists are professionally motivated to care for patients and willing to change their model of practice.	S W O T	
Pharmacists and technicians work well together as a team and respect each other's contributions to patient care.	S W O T	
The pharmacy has a sufficient number of staff to provide the current services.	S W O T	
Recruitment and retention efforts for pharmacy staff are not currently a problem.	S W O T	
Technicians are professionally motivated and willing to assume an expanded role in dispensing-related activities or other clinical support functions.	S W O T	
Pharmacy staff demonstrate professionalism in their work attitudes, patient interactions, behaviors, and appearance.	S W O T	
Policies and procedures are in place to facilitate staff recruitment, orientation, and discipline.	S W O T	
Pharmacists and technicians possess the appropriate interpersonal communication skills for establishing trusting relationships with patients and other providers.	S W O T	

continued on page 18

EXTERNAL DEMAND FACTORS

PATIENT CHARACTERISTICS	ANALYSIS	COMMENTS/NOTES
Patients typically seek out the pharmacist as a resource for health-related information.	S W O T	
Patients frequently convey concerns or have problems with their drug therapy.	S W O T	
Analysis of dispensing data indicates that drug use patterns are consistent with current or proposed patient services.	S W O T	
Analysis of prescribing patterns for specific conditions suggests drug therapy may be suboptimal.	S W O T	
Patients have sufficient household income to pay directly for services and frequently obtain alternative health services that they pay for out-of-pocket.	S W O T	
Patients belong to demographic groups that have been shown to seek health information and make informed choices about their medical treatment.	S W O T	
Patients conduct other personal business in the immediate service area or in the pharmacy.	S W O T	

EXTERNAL DEMAND FACTORS

PRESCRIBER & PROVIDER RELATIONS	ANALYSIS	COMMENTS/NOTES
Prescribers cooperate with the pharmacy in resolving prescription problems.	S W O T	
Prescribers are willing to discuss pharmacotherapy issues for specific patients and typically accept the pharmacist's recommendations for modifying therapy.	S W O T	
Prescribers frequently use the pharmacist as a source of drug information.	S W O T	
Prescribers initiate collaboration with the pharmacist to resolve individual patient problems related to drug therapy.	S W O T	

continued on page 19

EXTERNAL DEMAND FACTORS, continued

PRESCRIBER & PROVIDER RELATIONS	ANALYSIS	COMMENTS/NOTES
Prescribers have referred patients to the pharmacy for specific services/assistance.	S W O T	
The pharmacy engages in collaborative practice arrangements with prescribers or other health care providers to serve the needs of individual patients.	S W O T	
Other health care providers in the pharmacy's service area have requested assistance from the pharmacy on drug-related issues.	S W O T	
Potential exists to collaborate with other service providers who target patient groups with medical conditions known to pose drug therapy problems.	S W O T	
Mutual trust and respect exist between the pharmacy staff, prescribers, and other health care providers.	S W O T	

EXTERNAL DEMAND FACTORS

PAYER ENVIRONMENT	ANALYSIS	COMMENTS/NOTES
The pharmacy operates in an area where prescribers and hospitals participate in capitated reimbursement contracts.	S W O T	
The pharmacy operates in an area where third-party payers currently pay or are considering paying pharmacists for cognitive patient services.	S W O T	
The pharmacy operates in an area where potential exists for participating in demonstration projects funded by the pharmaceutical industry, third-party payers, or practice research initiatives.	S W O T	
The pharmacy operates in an area where employers typically self-fund their medical benefits for employees.	S W O T	

19

Chapter 2
CHANGING YOUR PRACTICE FOR PATIENT CARE
John P. Rovers & Jana M. Bajcar

Mark Pillar is the owner of Innovo-Medical Pharmacy, a large community pharmacy that sells gifts, cosmetics, toiletries, and greeting cards. It employs six pharmacists and six technicians. In recent years the pharmacy has added several well-received services: patient counseling, cholesterol checking, blood pressure monitoring, free home delivery, and diabetes disease management. Lately, however, profits are dropping. At the last staff meeting a new pharmacist, Grace Grady, suggested adding some disease management programs she saw presented at a professional meeting. Pharmacist Eric Benaround did not agree. Concerned that more services would not address the financial problems, he suggested that Mark think of ways to run the pharmacy more efficiently, including investing in robotic technology. A senior technician, Teresa Tecnique, wondered if they could attract more patients and increase revenue by improving customer service. Other pharmacists suggested trying to bring in more patients by offering monthly clinic days.

When the meeting ended, the discussion had not come to closure. Mark thanked everyone for their suggestions. "All your suggestions have merit," he said. "How about continuing this discussion at the next staff meeting?" Despite his upbeat tone, Mark left the meeting confused about how to proceed. Although he is committed to his patients and to enhancing the role of pharmacists, he wonders, "Where should I start?"

Change Is Necessary

Pharmacy managers and pharmacists across the country are in situations similar to Mark's. They are grappling with the many forces affecting today's health care settings—cost containment, redefined roles for health care professionals, competitors with advanced technology—and trying not to compromise the quality of patient care.

Like many pharmacists, Mark can see that his pharmacy must change if he wants to stay in business and keep serving his patients. Is that your situation, too? Whether you are in a community pharmacy, a primary care clinic, or a hospital pharmacy, do you recognize that your practice or department must refocus, but you don't know where to begin?

Although pharmacy managers who see the need for change try to respond productively, they often fail to consider a wide range of options. A hospital manager may visit colleagues at another institution, be impressed by their pharmacist-run anticoagulation clinic for ambulatory patients, and decide to launch a similar program. A community pharmacy manager may learn about a disease management program for asthma and launch one himself, or perhaps buy a franchise that includes patient care opportunities, such as specialty compounding. Once managers have decided on the new program, their typical route is to force it into the existing practice structure.

Sometimes this works, but often it doesn't. Either way, this approach has a key flaw: it is based on someone else's vision. It's risky to apply someone else's solution to your practice dilemma. You and your staff won't truly buy in to a new patient care program if it reflects the developer's values rather than your own. The program won't really be *yours*.

How will patients, physicians, and payers distinguish your practice from other pharmacies that acquire "one-size-fits-all" programs? Adding a new program is a good business decision only if it reflects your individual stamp and demonstrates to patients and physicians why they should use your pharmacy instead of another.

This chapter helps managers explore issues that arise and decisions to make after you realize you have to change, but before you have planned your new direction. It is best to dig into this material after completing the exercises suggested in Chapter 1, so you know what you want your practice to look like and have identified the values important to you. If you've done your homework first, whatever patient care program you choose will be *yours* and will reflect who you are as a professional.

Preparing to Change

Much of this chapter draws on the work of John Kotter,[1] a professor of management at the Harvard Business School. Academics and consultants who have tried to provoke change in pharmacy often have an "aha!" moment when reading Kotter's work because it makes clear why some pharmacies succeed and others fail. Although there is plenty of business literature that describes change, Kotter's approach is especially useful for the problems facing pharmacy.

Implementing Patient Care

+ Take stock of what your practice offers.
+ Explore the values underlying your practice.
+ Determine core motivators.
+ Create an image in your mind of the new practice.
+ Work through the eight steps for change (see box on page 30).

In *Leading Change*, Kotter states that "it is key to first establish your direction by developing your own vision of the desired future state." He adds that "without a sensible vision, a transformation effort can easily dissolve into a list of confusing and incompatible projects that can take the organization in the wrong direction or nowhere at all." For tools to help you take the first step in the change process—establishing your vision—see Step 2 in Chapter 1 (page 6) and pages 35–39 in this chapter.

Many authors of pharmacy literature voice the need for a clear direction and describe pharmacy practice models that could provide it. Some pharmacy practice models are:

 Develop a Vision

"It is key to first establish your direction by developing your own vision of the desired future state," says Harvard management professor John Kotter in his book *Leading Change*. "Without a sensible vision, a transformation effort can easily dissolve into a list of confusing and incompatible projects that can take the organization in the wrong direction or nowhere at all."

- **Total pharmacy care,**[2] which describes pharmacy practice as a combination of five subunits: distribution, self-care, drug information, clinical pharmacy, and pharmaceutical care.
- **Clinical pharmacy,**[3] a precursor to pharmaceutical care that has usually been practiced in institutional settings. Clinical pharmacists provide services that benefit patients, but the physician is the actual "client."
- **Pharmaceutical care,**[4] a successor to clinical pharmacy in which pharmacists take responsibility for patient outcomes. It is practiced in both institutional and community settings.
- **Disease management,**[5] which involves providing education and other clinical services to patients with specific diseases (such as asthma) or health goals (such as wanting to stop smoking).
- **Integrated pharmaceutical care service,**[6] which promotes pharmacists' responsibility for both patient care and drug product distribution.

Each model contributes in different ways to enhancing the role of the pharmacist and preparing the profession to meet the modern health care system's changing needs. But do they help Mark Pillar's situation in the case scenario described earlier?

Maybe, and maybe not. Although models described in the literature offer invaluable guidance, each group of practitioners needs to develop a shared vision of the future that is easy to communicate and is appealing to customers, stockholders, and employees.[1] Therefore, pharmacists must define how the model or philosophy fits into their practice. Kotter says that the vision need not be original; what is crucial is how well the vision serves users' interests and how easily it can be translated into a realistic, competitive strategy. Bad visions tend to ignore the legitimate needs and rights of important constituencies—favoring, say, employees over customers, he says.

Reflecting on Your Practice

✦ **Patients' perspective:** How do your patients feel about your pharmacy services? What do they see that makes your pharmacy different from others? Why do they patronize your pharmacy rather than the competition? What do they think you do well? What do they think you do badly?

✦ **Pharmacists' perspective:** What do your pharmacists do when they provide care or service to a patient? Do they all handle patients the same way? How is what they do similar and how is it different? What is the impact of the similarities and differences?

✦ **Health care providers' perspective:** What do physicians, nurses, and other providers experience when they ask a pharmacist a question? What do they experience when the pharmacist calls them to clarify a prescription order or discuss a patient's case?

✦ **Your perspective:** Do you have a clear idea of the values and principles that underlie your practice? Do you know what values you expect from your pharmacists?

Taking Stock of Your Practice

Ross Holland and Christine Nimmo, developers of the total pharmacy care model, point out that "many practitioners do not have a clear picture of how the new practice model is to fit into the current reality."[2] When developing a new direction, you must first take stock of your current practice. Define what it offers as well as the underlying values and principles. Describe it from different perspectives: patients, pharmacists, and other health care providers. Imagine how they would respond to the questions in the box to the left. If you are unsure what they would say, take time to ask them.

Values Underlying Change

For you to fully understand your practice you must explore the values and principles that underlie it. Are clear and consistent values at the foundation? Examples of these values may include:

✦ Offering high-quality patient service.
✦ Providing support and services to the health care team.
✦ Containing the rising drug budget.
✦ Providing care that respects the feelings and needs of patients.

You also must assess your personal values and principles regarding your practice, as well as those of your pharmacists and technicians. This may be more difficult than you think, mainly because people's actions sometimes demonstrate values that differ from the beliefs they espouse. For example, you may think you value the right of patients to participate in decisions about their medication-related care, yet when a patient intentionally stops adhering to the prescribed medication regimen you may react by lecturing about compliance. You may not take time to understand the patient's rationale for stopping the medication or to identify the assumptions that led the patient to his or her decision.

Identifying values takes effort and honesty. To figure out what values you and your pharmacists are conveying to others, talk with patients, pharmacists, and health care providers. The values they perceive may differ significantly from the ones you consider important.

Determining Core Motivators

To identify the new environment you'd like in your pharmacy or department—built on your chosen values and principles—you must determine core factors that motivate your pharmacists and technicians in their daily tasks. These factors fall into three broad categories: business and economics, service, and care (see sidebar on page 25). Although clear connections exist among these motivators, you must decide which will take precedence in your vision of a new practice. Then choose the values or principles that underlie the vision.

The categories overlap and are synergistic. Providing quality care or service can be good for business, but if the primary motivator underlying a practice is business, service or care will not automatically result. When thinking about what "service" means, a useful analogy is a waiter in a restaurant. Customers

Because Mark can't fully answer the questions in the sidebar on page 23, he takes time to speak with some customers while they wait for their prescriptions. He has coffee with his pharmacists and technicians. He visits a few local physicians. Through this process he gets a realistic view of his pharmacy practice.

The first things patients see when entering the pharmacy, he learns, are cashiers at their registers and staff offering help with selecting cosmetics or merchandise. At the pharmacy counter, patients are met by a technician who gathers information about their drug plans and receives the prescription order. Then patients usually must wait 20 minutes to see a pharmacist, who briefly describes how the medication should be taken and provides written information. Pharmacists offer some patients cholesterol or blood pressure checks. Next, patients pay the pharmacist for the medication.

Meetings with the pharmacists reveal similarities and differences in how they approach their patient practice. Some pharmacists first review the prescription order for completeness and compare it to the medication profile to pinpoint potential drug interactions. They pass it to the technician for filling and then meet with the patient to review the directions. Other pharmacists start by reviewing the medication profile. Then they verify key information with the patient and, if this points to problems, they contact the physician before having the technician fill the prescription. When they talk to the patient, they go beyond reviewing directions. They determine the patient's understanding of medications being dispensed that day and provide education to enable him or her to take the medications properly.

continued on page 25

Mark Finds Variations in Practice

continued from page 24

Some physicians Mark interviews say that pharmacists from his pharmacy call them only to check unclear handwriting. Others say pharmacists call to suggest therapy modifications or to bring to their attention new information that could affect a patient's care. Mark learns that some of his pharmacists, but not all, give patients blood pressure and cholesterol measurements to take to their physicians. Some physicians say that their diabetic patients have received wonderful, comprehensive care from certain pharmacists.

Clearly, Mark's pharmacy practice looks different from the three perspectives and there are differences in how each pharmacist approaches practice.

Motivating Factors

* **Business and economics:** These factors include cost-containment, market share, revenue, profits, and the pharmacy's viability to stay in business.

* **Service:** This has to do with competently delivering services that patients or health care providers want. Examples of pharmacy services include drug information, pharmacokinetic dosing, anticoagulant dosing, intravenous additive programs, disease management services, and drug distribution.

* **Care:** The essence of care is honoring patients, respecting their feelings and needs, and helping them to be heard.

choose what they want, with or without suggestions from the waiter. Even if the waiter offers opinions about the menu, his or her role is to process the customer's request accurately, competently, efficiently, and courteously.

Different definitions have been proposed for "care," a term that has recently received much attention in the nursing and pharmacy literature.[7] This book reflects the definition put forth by nursing consultants Denise Lillian Hawthorne and Nancy Jane Yurkovich[8]: "Caring is an act of accepting, enabling and encouraging an individual by honoring his uniqueness, his complexity, his feelings and needs; by believing that each person's life makes a difference; and by helping a person find his voice and be heard." The pharmaceutical care philosophy captures the essence of care because it focuses primarily on patients and not drugs, promotes a therapeutic relationship between patients and pharmacists, involves patients in their care, considers all the patient's drug-related needs, and seeks to achieve positive outcomes.[4]

Although service and care are different, each has a role in pharmacy practice, according to Holland and Nimmo.[2] Still, it is essential that service functions be recognized as such and not be confused with care. Otherwise the new direction you set may not be clear to yourself or to the people you want to follow you.

Pharmacists must reflect honestly on the three following questions to determine where to start implementing change and whether the primary motivator will be service or care.

1. What do you do when you provide service to a customer?
2. What do you do when you provide care to a patient?
3. How are these two activities different, and how are they similar?

One of the biggest differences between providing service to customers and providing care to patients is the degree to which you accept responsibility. The idea of accepting complete responsibility for medication-related care of patients can be both scary and, in many situations, not realistic. To provide care, you must be aware of your abilities and parameters of responsibility. You must also recognize the extent to which you can accept responsibility for care-related activities (see sidebar on page 27). To a large degree, the practice site dictates the amount of responsibility you can accept, although pharmacists in all settings should be able to accept responsibility for patients' understanding of and adherence to drug therapy. Think about what you *can* be responsible for—not just what you *want* to be responsible for—and then accept those responsibilities.

When providing care to patients, pharmacists also provide clinical services such as drug information, drug therapy monitoring, pharmacokinetic dosing, and disease management programs. But does providing the available services automatically translate to providing care? Probably not. Services can be a stepping stone to providing care—but only if you

CASE EXAMPLE:
Varied Values at Innovo-Medical

If Mark were to try identifying a common set of values among his pharmacists and technicians, patients would probably say that all the staff are respectful, friendly, and eager to help. Physicians would say something similar. Still, Mark would be unclear about the values and principles that underlie these behaviors. As he and his staff undertake the change process described later in this chapter, Mark will need to keep in mind that, right now, neither he nor his staff are fully aware of the values behind what they do.

The suggestions his staff members made earlier suggest that they espouse different values, including business and economics (Eric) and service (Grace). When Mark establishes his guiding coalition (described in Step 2, page 32) he will want to make sure these diverse views are represented. That way, staff members can hash out their thoughts to develop a practice vision shared by all.

Definition of Care

"Caring is an act of accepting, enabling and encouraging an individual by honoring his uniqueness, his complexity, his feelings and needs; by believing that each person's life makes a difference; and by helping a person find his voice and be heard."

Source: Hawthorne DL. Yurkovich NJ. Caring: the essence of health care professions. Human Health Care International. 1996;12(1):27-8

Accepting Responsibility

What can pharmacists accept responsibility for when providing care to patients? Some possible answers to this question include making sure that patients:

+ Understand their medications.
+ Adhere with prescribed medications.
+ Are on the best medications for their condition.

Answers will vary among practitioners and practice sites. But instead of asking whether pharmacists can accept *full* responsibility for these activities, it would be better to ask *to what extent* pharmacists can accept responsibility. When cast this way, the answer depends on such factors as whether the pharmacist practices in a team-based model or as an independent practitioner, the pharmacist's knowledge and skills, and support structures that help or hinder the pharmacist's ability to be accountable. In other words, a pharmacist in a high-volume chain pharmacy probably can't take responsibility for routinely helping physicians choose medications for diabetes patients, but a pharmacist in a diabetes clinic can.

understand the difference between the two. You consciously decide to use services to move toward care.

Creating an Image

After taking stock of your practice and determining your principal motivating factor, you must create an image in your mind of the new pharmacy practice you want to develop. Do this from multiple perspectives—those of patients, pharmacists, and other health care providers. Gather information from the literature about models of practice or visit sites that have implemented new practices. The total pharmacy care model,[2] for example, integrates five existing pharmacy practice models—drug information, self-care, clinical pharmacy, pharmaceutical care, and distribution—and helps you analyze which are key motivating factors.

Implementing Your New Patient Care Program

This section, which helps you develop a plan for changing your practice, draws further on John Kotter's ideas. His book *Leading Change*[1] identifies an eight-stage process you must follow to create change (see box on page 30).

Although you may do several steps simultaneously, it is vital that you address them all thoroughly, in the order presented. And be patient. You may have some fast successes, but it will probably take several years before you can be sure that a change is in place and that your pharmacists have genuinely taken it into their hearts.

Your staff may not be able to implement the new vision as fast as the marketplace demands. This will be frustrating, but it's something you must accept. By the time pharmacists enter practice they've already acquired certain skills and knowledge and have developed attitudes about who they are, what they do, what they expect from the workplace, and what the workplace expects from them. Creating changes that pharmaceutical care demands means asking pharmacists to reorient who they are and what they do. The human psyche allows people to change only so fast.

Similarly, your organization likely has dozens of policies, procedures, and "that's the way we do things around here" items that may slow your progress. Your leadership, patience, and ability to tolerate staff members' struggles will be a major asset as you implement your new patient care program.

Step 1: Establish a Sense of Urgency

Do most pharmacists feel an urgent need to change their practices soon? Consultants, college faculty, and others leading the profession's pharmaceutical care movement say the answer is no. Pharmacists have shown amazing resourcefulness in dealing with recent challenges, such as chronic staff shortages. Most marginal operators have been driven out of the community pharmacy business in the past decade, and the survivors have been able to maintain economically viable practices despite declining reimbursements. It is predicted that prescription volumes will increase by 5% to 12% annually over the next five years,[9]

CASE EXAMPLE:
Mark's Motivators

Mark's response to his staff's suggestions will depend on whether he is motivated by business, service, or care values. If he is primarily motivated by business, then Eric's suggestions about efficiency and technology may seem most relevant. If Mark is primarily motivated by service, Grace's idea about new disease management programs may be more useful. However, if Mark's motivation is care, he may wonder if any of the suggestions will help move the pharmacy practice toward his vision.

Mark needs to determine how to use a service as a stepping stone to providing care. Suppose, for example, that Grace had suggested implementing a flu shot program each fall. To turn this service into care—so it's not just like the flu shot programs offered by other pharmacies—Mark must see that the service reflects the individual needs of patients as well as the responsibility taken by the pharmacist. Mark would start this transition by using the pharmacy's database to identify patients at high risk for the flu. Instead of simply posting a sign in the pharmacy, he'd inform high-risk patients individually that the pharmacy is reserving vaccine specifically for them. Mark would explain that vaccine will not be released to the general public until the needs of high-risk patients are met. So although Mark would be offering flu shots (a service), accepting responsibility for identifying high-risk patients would turn the service into care.

CASE EXAMPLE:
What Would Mark Do?

If, using the total pharmacy care model, Mark decides the primary motivating factor is business, then he may emphasize making profits from drug distribution and self-care. If he decides it's care, then he may place priority on developing and integrating all five aspects of the total pharmacy care model. If Mark's primary factor is service, he may focus on fast, cheap, friendly service and customer satisfaction.

What to Accomplish Before Going Further

The rest of this chapter builds on material in other parts of the book, including the first half of this chapter. Before applying what you are about to read, you must:

+ Develop a detailed idea of the patient care programs you wish to launch. Chapters 5 and 6 give information on finding such programs and getting the necessary training.

+ Ground your patient care programs in the values espoused by you and your organization.

+ Define your unique philosophy of practice, which reflects your values.

+ Meet with patients and physicians associated with your practice to determine their needs and decide how you can meet them.

+ Review and purchase any commercially available programs you want to use. Chapters 6 lists organizations that offer such programs.

which gives a certain measure of comfort. Although the margin per prescription is dropping, the total volume of prescriptions filled should allow practices to survive.

The same is true in health systems. Hospital pharmacists have survived what must have seemed like an endless stream of consultants who reviewed their practices and recommended adding technology and downsizing staff. As for individual pharmacists, the outlook is rosy. The current shortage means that any pharmacist looking for a job will find one with minimal effort, earn a generous salary, and possibly receive a signing bonus.

Life under managed care may not be wonderful, but pharmacy organizations continue to function, pharmacies remain profitable, and most pharmacists are well paid for their work. After listening to doomsday scenarios for a decade, pharmacists are still here. The attitude of many is, "We've come through a difficult period and we're tired. You want us to change again? No way!"

This attitude is your first challenge as a manager trying to get pharmacists to embrace a new practice model. They may feel that there isn't much reason to change at this point. So you must help your staff recognize the need for change and establish a sense of urgency to propel your organization forward.

Ask your pharmacists how technology will affect the nature of their work. What will the future be like once dispensing robots are cheap enough to be widely available? Some may not have considered being replaced by machines. Careers of some hospital pharmacists have been disrupted by technology, but the demand for pharmacists elsewhere has been strong enough to absorb those downsized out of a job. But what if three or four national chains employing 20,000 pharmacists were to replace half their staff with robots or central fill dispensing programs? That would mean 10,000 pharmacists dumped into the marketplace at once. Do your pharmacists think their particular skills will make them valuable in such a scenario? If most of their job skills relate strictly to filling prescriptions, will they be able to compete for jobs?

 Eight Steps for Change

Below are John Kotter's eight steps for creating change.[1] If you omit any, change their order, or do them haphazardly, he says, your change effort will fail.

1. Establish a sense of urgency.
2. Create the guiding coalition.
3. Develop a vision and strategy.
4. Communicate the change vision.
5. Empower broad-based action.
6. Generate short-term wins.
7. Consolidate gains and produce more change.
8. Anchor new approaches in the culture.

A key effect of technology has been the creation of a knowledge-based economy that needs workers with skills in collaborative problem-solving, communication, teamwork, managing information, and dealing with uncertainty. A major change in your practice can provide your pharmacists the opportunity to develop their skills in these increasingly important areas. Remind your staff that the ability to think is a skill employers will always be willing to buy in a knowledge-based economy.

Another way to create a sense of urgency is to consider your pharmacists' satisfaction. Recent information suggests that many pharmacists are not satisfied with the quality of their work life.[10] If a pharmacist's dissatisfaction stems from frustration at not being able to function as professionally as she wants, a savvy manager could tout change as an opportunity for her to reclaim her professional identity. The workplace may still present frustrations that impede change, but if the changes that take place improve the pharmacist's self image, her motivation for change will increase.

You can also appeal to pharmacists' sense of professionalism and social responsibility. Because pharmacists view themselves as health care professionals, most will do the right thing for the right reason if given the means and opportunity. Tap into their sense of humanity and their basic human need to be valued and appreciated. Once a pharmacist knows what it feels like to truly care for a patient and to receive heartfelt gratitude from the patient or physician, it's hard to revert back to a dispensing-only mode. Most pharmacists feel rewarded for making a difference and alleviat-

CASE EXAMPLE:
Mark's Staff Wants Change

During initial discussions, Mark learns that many of his pharmacists are only partially satisfied with their jobs. They take pride in their patient care activities, but spend most of their time dispensing drugs. Although they are busy, they find the routines of their practice boring.

One day pharmacist Eric tells Mark that he just filled several prescriptions for Greta Gasp, a patient the pharmacy has regularly provided with inhalers to relieve her asthma. She gave Eric a whole slew of new prescriptions for inhalers and tablets to prevent asthma attacks and for a steroid to be taken when her asthma worsens. She told Eric that she spent the night in the emergency room with a severe asthma attack. Mark and Eric review Greta's profile and notice that refills for her asthma reliever have been growing in frequency the past two months. Mark recognizes that his staff is looking for new challenges, and that a patient might have avoided an emergency room visit if the pharmacy had offered an asthma program to prevent poor outcomes.

Using published data about medication-use problems from the Institute of Medicine and other sources, Mark starts casual discussions with his staff about the need for change. They express a desire for change and offer suggestions about ways to do it. This is great, because it means the push for change will come from Mark's staff, not from him.

ing human suffering. Help them understand that this feeling can be part of their everyday work lives. Sure, there will always be patients who take out their frustrations on pharmacists, but such unpleasantness shrinks in importance when pharmacists have the sense of dignity and self-worth that comes from functioning as a true health care professional.

Patients' problems with drug therapy and the consequences of these problems have become increasingly clear in recent years. The cost of drug therapy problems is now estimated at over $76 billion.[11] The report *To Err Is Human* published by the Institute of Medicine shows that up to 94,000 Americans die from medical errors each year and that many of these errors are related to drug therapy.[12] That's the equivalent of a fully loaded Boeing 747 crashing every two days. Making your staff aware of these statistics can increase their sense of urgency. Although pharmacists' role in causing or preventing errors is not fully clear, it's evident that the high rate of medical errors presents pharmacists with an opportunity to significantly improve public health.

Consider doing detective work in your practice to uncover a patient whose outcome from drug therapy was poor—an outcome that could have been different if your pharmacy had embraced a new practice model. Most pharmacists on your staff will be sufficiently professional to want to prevent such problems and to create a practice environment that lets them.

Step 2: Create the Guiding Coalition

Usually the combined efforts of a few dedicated, talented people drive change, not one dynamic leader who directs events from the top. Thus, you must put together a team to bring about change.

If you work in an organized health care setting you're probably thinking, "Oh no, not another committee! How will I get people to agree to this?" But if you've presented a convincing case for change, staff will be enthusiastic about helping.

If you're in a small community you may wonder how to create a team when your employees consist of two pharmacists and a technician. The team's size and its makeup will depend on the size of the practice, the complexity of programs to be developed, and the staff's level of interest in the proposed change. Sometimes a team may have only two or three members. The take-home message is that owners and managers should not be the sole driving force for change.

The most important condition—one that seems to predict the success or failure of any change coalition—is having a blend of *leaders* and *managers.* In the sense used here, these terms represent personal styles, not job titles. *Managers* are the more common of the two. Management is a skill that can be taught and involves placing controls on an organization so it functions smoothly and predictably. *Managers* oversee budgets, staffing, policies, procedures, and inventory and create systems that help the organization reach its goals. Determining what those goals are is not something that *managers* necessarily do well.

Leadership is a trait that probably can't be taught. *Leaders* determine the organization's goals and tell everyone on staff where they are going. Whereas management places controls, organizes, and solves problems, leadership establishes direction, motivates, and inspires. Effective leadership results in an energized staff eager to change, grow, and improve.

On teams with a good blend, *leaders* provide the inspiration and direction. *Managers* keep everybody on task and ensure that all pieces are in place to create a new practice model.

Key Strategies for Sparking Urgency

+ Attune pharmacists to the benefits of having marketable skills in a knowledge-based economy.
+ Tap into staff's desires for more professional satisfaction.
+ Appeal to pharmacists' sense of social responsibility and their need to be valued.
+ Highlight an example in your practice that shows how proposed changes could have helped a patient avoid a severe health problem or hospitalization.

Who Should Be Part of Your Guiding Coalition?

Below are things to consider when creating the team that will guide your organization toward change.

Position power. Does your coalition include pharmacists and non-pharmacists who have the power to either drive change forward or block it? If the staff believes that the group guiding change does not include members powerful enough to make something happen, they are unlikely to take the process seriously. Depending on your organization's size, consider appointing some members from the very highest levels of management. A district supervisor for a chain pharmacy or a hospital vice-president known to support the proposed change will send a strong message to staff about how seriously the organization takes the change effort.

Expertise. Does your team include people with a variety of skills and job descriptions? Does it have the expertise to make decisions wisely? Does it include some pharmacists who are patient care experts and others who are experts on the health care system? Are some members hard-nosed quantitative types, while others are more sensitive to the impact proposed changes will have on staff, other health care providers, and patients? Create a pool of talent that is as broad and deep as your practice will allow.

continued on page 34

All members of the team should already feel the urgency described in the previous section. They must also be able to trust each other. If, for example, a technician on the team suspects that the pharmacists are merely trying to dump work on her and her colleagues, meaningful change is unlikely to occur. Organizations that do not have a culture of mutual trust and respect may need to do team-building exercises or take part in off-site retreats with an experienced external consultant. The local office of the Small Business Administration or a nearby business school may be able to recommend a team-building consultant.

Whether you use a consultant or not, building trust requires that pharmacy staff get together (preferably off site) and air their concerns. Establish ground rules first, such as, "It's okay to attack ideas and actions, but not people."

When an organization has a deeply ingrained culture of mistrust, staff members want to be heard. Your role at first is simply to listen. Don't talk, don't explain, and don't defend. This may be difficult, but your staff needs the chance to blow off steam. Once concerns have been openly voiced, you can explore whether any are based on misperceptions, misinformation, or unrealistic expectations.

Look for common threads. If more than one staff member is upset about something, it's probably a major issue to them all. Don't expect to resolve all the concerns in one meeting. What's most important is for staff to be convinced that management is listening and is serious about making things better. After your initial information-gathering meeting, you can develop plans for change that address the issues raised.

CASE EXAMPLE:
Mark's Guiding Coalition

As Mark creates his guiding coalition he realizes that he must be the leader, even though this makes him uncomfortable. He will depend on others for fine-tuning, but right now he is the only one with a general vision for the practice's new direction. He invites pharmacists Eric and Grace to join the team. Both have different personalities and views, and both are highly respected by their peers. Eric, with his interest in management and his quantitative skills, will act as manager for the change process to ensure realistic goals and smooth functioning. He tends to be skeptical, but once he's convinced of something he follows through on it. Grace will be a good representative for pharmacists seeking new challenges. Although she is more focused on service than care, Mark thinks she will easily make the mental transition between the two once she grasps the differences.

Who Should Be Part of Your Guiding Coalition? continued

Credibility. How are the members of your team viewed by their colleagues? Will some members be viewed as "political appointees" who will not necessarily contribute much to the team's progress? If members are unthinkingly and uniformly supportive of the manager or organization, the team will lack credibility.

Leadership. Does your team include both *managers* and *leaders*? Too many *leaders* can result in a lot of grand, impractical plans. Too many *managers* can slow the process, because management focuses on making operations smooth and predictable.

Mark also includes technician Dee Spence, partly to represent technicians and partly because she's considered a "handful" to manage. If Dee does not want something to happen, she can enlist most of the technicians and pharmacists to help her block it. Mark knows that Dee's support, vital to their success, is much more likely if she has been part of the planning process.

Mark also asks two outsiders to join the coalition to ensure that interests beyond those of the pharmacy are represented. He invites Nurse Liz, who works for a local physician with whom Mark is friendly. He would love to have the physician on the team, but knows that the nurse has more flexibility to attend meetings. He will depend on Nurse Liz to carry ideas, objections, and suggestions between the pharmacy and the physician (who, Mark hopes, will talk with medical colleagues about the pharmacy's planned changes, giving Nurse Liz even more input).

Finally, Mark invites Greta Gasp to represent patients' concerns. Greta has multiple health problems, takes several medications, and is confident and articulate.

Step 3: Develop a Vision and Strategy

Because pharmacists are professionally socialized to be careful, cautious, detail-oriented, and quantitative in their thinking, the concept of "vision" may make them uncomfortable. They may view it as a vague, fuzzy concept—something that can't be measured. A vision for change is not part of pharmacists' professional vocabulary. (For more information about creating a vision, see Chapter 1, page 6.)

Instead of operating from the standpoint of vision, especially in organized health care settings, pharmacists usually manage change by creating policies and procedures or job descriptions that describe what has to be done, who is going to do it, and how it should be carried out. Although change can happen when it is micromanaged this way, progress will be slow and few people will feel inspired. Well-developed policies and procedures are necessary, but in and of themselves are unlikely to result in much change. (See Chapters 4, 5, and 6 for information on creating policies and procedures and human resource tools that support a vision for change.)

A few pharmacies may have leaders who can cause change through sheer force of personality (or even outright bullying), but more than likely staff will find a way to subvert change that is driven this way. Attempting to bring about change by decree from the top or by closely managing details does not usually work. Change that stems from a shared vision *does* work.

The blend of managerial and leadership talent on your guiding coalition will create your vision for change. The *leader* types generally create the vision and some strategies for achieving it. The *manager* types develop detailed plans and budgets to implement the strategies. If the vision involves providing care to diabetic patients, for example, the required strategies will probably include training staff. *Managers* will determine exactly who needs to be trained, how and when to train them, and what resources to allocate.

Features of a Vision

Don't confuse a "vision" with a mission statement. Mission statements tell the public who you are, what you do, and what they can expect. They do not indicate where you are going and what you want your organization to be. A good mission statement can help you achieve your vision, but it does not necessarily describe that vision.

A well-phrased vision of your practice is an internal document; you do not necessarily share it with the public. It describes what you want your future to be like, tells your staff where they are going, and coordinates efforts. If confusion occurs or arguments come up about an idea during the change process, you can check your vision statement for clarification. When change is painful, a clear vision can reassure people and remind them why it is desirable to achieve a certain goal. Some organizations already have vision statements. Those with the characteristics in the box on page 36 can be useful for driving change.

Good Vision Statements

Vision statements that are useful for driving change tend to have these characteristics:

+ **A description that is imaginable.** If your staff can't see what a practice will be like based on your vision, you need to go back and try again. If your vision is "to be the pharmacy of the future," don't be surprised if nobody knows what you're talking about. Such a vision is too vague to imagine clearly.

+ **A scope that meets the needs of everyone your practice touches.** If your new vision awards most of the advantages to only one of the groups your practice involves—patients, families, physicians, nurses, staff—and dumps most of the disadvantages on another, rewrite the vision to describe a future that all the groups will find desirable.

+ **Feasibility.** Your vision needs to describe a future sufficiently different from the present to make your staff stretch to meet it. Goals that can be reached with no effort and at little cost will not transform the practice. Challenge your staff. But at the same time, make sure your goals are achievable. Those that are not, simply cause frustration. Setting a balance between a challenging vision and an unrealistic one is a delicate task. Of course, even an achievable vision can seem impossible to staff, so draw on your leadership skills to encourage them. Keep the focus on the positive aspects of the vision and on the urgent need for change.

+ **A balance of focus and detail.** A good vision is well focused, but not so detailed that it becomes inflexible. For example, if you make the vague statement that you want to "be the best," how will you know when you've achieved the vision? By the same token, if your vision is exhaustively detailed, you won't be able to fine-tune it as circumstances change.

+ **Ability to be communicated.** Your vision must be worded simply enough for everyone involved to understand, but not so childishly written as to lack credibility. The proper wording may depend on whether you will be communicating your vision to nonpharmacists and people outside the pharmacy staff. For those groups, pharmacy jargon and "insider" terminology are inappropriate.

If you are a pharmacist guided by the vision on page 37 you should be able to see the practice clearly. You can imagine yourself dealing primarily with patients and meeting the needs of all stakeholders in the pharmacy. Patients receive good care. Physicians and nurses are aided in their work. Staff are valued and proud of their good reputations. Owners and stockholders receive any additional profits.

The goal of providing screening services to every patient is a stretch; staff will see it as a challenge. That's okay, because the intention is to transform practice rather than maintain the status quo.

The statement is focused but flexible enough to allow for a variety of care services. Finally, it is easy to read and can be understood readily by staff. Perhaps a multipage, detailed description could back up the vision and describe the implementation process, but the statement itself is short and easy to communicate. It is also free of jargon so that patients and others outside the practice can understand it.

Step 4: Communicate the Change Vision

The challenge now is to get the vision out to the organization and let staff examine it and ask questions. This can be a time of both discussion and reflection as everyone in the pharmacy begins to understand the new vision's impact on them.

CASE EXAMPLE:
Vision Statement

After much discussion, Mark and his coalition develop the following vision statement:

"By the end of 2005, we will become the pharmacy of choice for patients who value care and service more than they value inexpensive prescriptions. We will change our focus from dispensing prescriptions to caring for people. Our reputation for care and competence will motivate patients to seek us out. Other health care professionals will want us to work with them to ensure that medications they prescribe have the intended effects. Our pharmacists, technicians, and support staff will be proud of our practice and their role in it. Each patient who comes to the pharmacy will be screened to detect problems with his/her drug therapy. Patients who have problems will be offered appropriate patient care services. Through our daily actions, we will demonstrate our value in the health care system and we will make every effort to seek reasonable compensation for our work."

Staff will ask themselves if they agree with the new vision, whether they can make the changes needed to support it, whether they want to support it, and what alternatives there may be to the vision. They will be deeply concerned with determining the vision's impact on them, their jobs, and their workplace—and their fears about change may make the vision hard to absorb. If you do not communicate the vision properly, it will damage your chances for successful change.

Keep the message simple. If your vision for change includes the jargon pharmacists use when talking to each other—drug therapy problems, outcomes, pharmaceutical care, etc.—nonpharmacists interested in your vision won't understand it.

Use analogies, metaphors, and similes to illustrate the vision. A phrase like "we'll care for patients as if we were their mothers" may sound hokey, but its intention is clear to practically anyone.

Communicate your vision to your staff in multiple ways, on multiple days. An article or two in the pharmacy's newsletter or an announcement at a staff meeting are not enough. Think about how much news, data, and gossip staff are exposed to daily. Messages about the vision can easily get buried in torrents of other information. Use your guiding coalition and your management team—which should be two different entities—to promote the vision daily and educate people about its components.

Creating the Vision

Usually, the leaders on your guiding coalition—who are likely to have the clearest view of the new practice—will create the first draft of the vision. The draft should describe the leaders' dreams for the new practice and how they envision it fitting into the health care system and marketplace. The rest of the guiding coalition should review the first draft, test it in practice, and suggest changes. This step may take the coalition considerable time, discussion, and soul-searching. Don't be surprised if the process is messy at times or leads to heated debate. If you have chosen your guiding coalition well, members will trust each other enough to work through differences.

A good vision for change will not be written in a single meeting or in a few days. Occasional off-site retreats may be necessary to work out points of contention. In the end, the vision should give staff a clear goal to reach and should be something the pharmacy's owners, managers, department heads, and administrators can agree on. The vision's overall purpose is to transform the practice.

Each time you consider hiring someone, check to see how well he or she fits into the new vision. Communicating your philosophy of practice before new employees come on board helps you pinpoint and avoid potential conflicts in ideology.

If you change the staff schedule, ask whether the new shifts help staff understand and implement the new vision. During performance appraisals, include feedback regarding staff's contributions to the vision's success. Every conversation with your staff is an opportunity to promote your new practice.

Pharmacy administrators must demonstrate their commitment to the vision

Conveying the Vision to Staff

- Keep the message simple and avoid jargon.
- Use analogies, metaphors, and similes to illustrate the vision.
- Communicate your vision in multiple ways, on multiple days.
- When hiring new people, select those who buy in to the vision.
- Make sure that pharmacy leaders demonstrate their commitment to the vision.
- Keep mixed messages to a minimum.
- Encourage feedback.

CASE EXAMPLE:
Mark's Coalition Gets Out the Message

Mark's coalition decides that a combination of words and actions will get out the message most effectively. They start conducting themselves in accordance with the vision as part of their daily routine. When pharmacists Grace and Eric refill prescriptions, they ask patients screening questions to uncover possible drug therapy problems. Through their efforts, they identify two or three problems each day that require clinical skill to solve. The other pharmacists notice these changes.

Technician Dee starts inviting patients to sit down and discuss their drug therapy with a pharmacist—and the other technicians notice. Grace, Eric, and Dee discuss their actions with coworkers, answer their questions, and gather feedback on the new practice model. Everyone begins to see how the new practice fits into the existing structure. They recognize that it is both useful to patients and doable by pharmacists and technicians.

Mark discusses the new vision at a staff meeting. Because he knows that a single mention is unlikely to stick with the staff, he also has a series of one-on-one meetings to educate everyone who works in the pharmacy and hear their thoughts. Over the next few months, every time he conveys a management decision he asks how well his managerial changes help staff embrace the new vision. Six months after distributing the vision statement, Mark is confident that everyone on staff has a basic understanding of the new practice.

each day. When promoting people, choose those who support the vision for change. Do not allow anyone to avoid the discomfort caused by change (such as a shift supervisor who tries to delegate all "unpleasant" duties to others).

Although mixed messages will be unavoidable at times, keep them to a minimum. Sometimes you may need to act in ways that the staff views as inconsistent with the change message. For example, you may be emphasizing patient care at the same time that upper management is about to contract with a third-party payer that focuses on price. In cases like this, be honest with your staff. Explain the reasons why a mixed message is being sent. Reemphasize the vision's importance and outline how you, as the pharmacy manager, will deal with upper level administration. Let them know you will go all out to support their patient care efforts. Some staff members may be skeptical, but they will appreciate your honesty. Keep any promises you make, or you will damage your credibility as a change leader.

Because communication is a two-way street, encourage staff to provide feedback about the vision's appropriateness and the progress being made towards its implementation. Although your guiding coalition has devoted a great deal of energy to developing a vision for change, it is conceivable that they got it wrong. The time you spend listening may slow the pace of change, but it may save considerable effort if it prevents problems that could arise from a less-than-ideal vision.

Step 5: Empower Broad-Based Action

"Empowering" your employees may sound complicated, but it really means simply taking the weight of the organization off their backs so they can launch the changes desired in the new practice. Most of the previous steps have focused on producing change in individuals. This one examines structural changes in the organization that allow staff to change.

Four types of barriers generally impede an employee's ability to cooperate with a vision for change: structural, educational, systems-related, and supervisory.

Structural Barriers

What structural barriers could hinder change in your hospital or pharmacy? Although at first glance, your answer may be "none," look more closely. Do the health care teams in your environment operate as effectively as possible? Pharmacists will need to work with physicians and nurses under your new practice model. You may need the cooperation of other departments: social work, laboratory, and radiology, for example. Is this new or threatening for other practitioners? If so, you will need to remove this barrier.

Organizations tend to form into structural silos. Improvements in one silo are usually perceived as occurring at the expense of another—a perception you will need to address if it's inherent in your institution. For instance, if your new practice includes taking medication histories, nursing staff may think you are encroaching on their status and responsibilities. Physicians may believe that pharmacists offering consulting services jeopardize their own consults with patients and medical colleagues. To avoid the "silo" mentality, be prepared to demonstrate how your changes can benefit others in the organization. You might, for example, show nurses that pharmacists' drug histories are more complete, which makes them more useful for everyone. You could explain to physicians that your consulting service focuses on patient education, not on diagnosis or drug selection, and therefore, is not an economic threat.

Not all pharmacists have mutually respectful, cooperative relationships with local physicians. And some situations permit only the traditional doctor-pharmacist relationship. If local physicians do not think of you as a colleague—or if they see themselves in one silo, you in another—it can interfere with practice changes. Critically examine the relationships you will need as you change your practice. Ensure that lines of communication are open and that a spirit of cooperation exists or is being developed.

Tell local physicians about the changes you are planning. Explain that their support will be helpful, but do not come across as if you are seeking their permission. Meet with physician colleagues when you can; try to arrange an invitation to address the local medical association about your changes. Although some physicians are sure to object to your proposed changes, and may even make you feel uncomfortable, it's a great opportunity to identify their objections (such as, "You're not qualified to do that") and to address them (by outlining the additional training staff will receive, for example).

Within the pharmacy itself there may be structural barriers to change. As pharmacists start making patient care decisions in the new practice, supervisors may react negatively if a subordinate's decision is poor or controversial. Will supervisors support pharmacists when physicians do not agree with their actions or when they perceive an intervention as ill-considered? Pharmacists who see their new practice continually second-guessed or not supported by supervisors will start to wonder why they should embrace the changes. Modifying the reporting structures between managers and pharmacists may be necessary to better handle disagreements about patient care issues.

Educational Barriers

Your pharmacists may not have all the necessary patient care skills for the new practice and may need training to address gaps in knowledge, skills, and attitudes. (See Chapter 6 for information on staff development issues.)

Systems-Related Barriers

Barriers related to human resources, information systems, and drug distribution may impede change. How well are the motivational and incentives systems in your pharmacy aligned with your desired change? If you are changing to a patient-focused practice, but a manager's year-end bonus depends on prescription volume, you can't expect people to devote more effort to patient care. Another example of a systems barrier is determining staffing solely by distribution workload—that is, by the volume of tasks related to preparing and dispensing medications—rather than by patient care workload.

What types of information will your pharmacists need to change the practice? How will they obtain it and what will they do with it? Do you need to develop relationships with local physicians so they will cooperate in providing information about individual patients? Should you create a medical information release form for patients to sign so that physicians will share necessary information? Do pharmacists have computer access to laboratory and clinical data? Is a system in place for documenting patient information? Do you need permission to write in medical charts? Must the pharmacy buy or develop its own documentation system? The answer to each of these questions could uncover a potential systems barrier.

To deal with distribution barriers, you must examine how your drug distribution system functions and ensure that pharmacists' job descriptions and responsibilities reflect patient care rather than dispensing. How must the distribution system be modi-

41

fied to allow time for patient care? Be certain that appropriate nonclinical tasks are delegated to adequately trained technicians.

Supervisory Barriers

The final step in empowering staff for change is making sure that supervisory personnel do not consciously or unconsciously inhibit change. Supervisors, usually your most senior and trusted personnel, may have political connections to people above you in the organization. Some supervisors can be a threat if they have the ear of higher-ups and want to block your changes.

CASE EXAMPLE:
Mark's Staff Pinpoints Changes

At this point Mark and his staff identify exactly what needs to be changed and how. They look at staffing, training, marketing, and pharmacy workflow and plug specific tasks into a table like that in Figure 1-1 (page 12). Then they determine who is responsible for each task and the deadline by which it must be completed. Everyone in the pharmacy is given responsibilities to help bring about change.

Although such problems are unpleasant, ignoring them gives a mixed message to your staff. Start by talking with supervisors about the proposed direction and asking about their concerns. Explore whether their concerns are with the actual vision (what you are trying to change) or with the process (how you are trying to implement the change). They may have useful alternative perspectives that address a missing piece in your plan. They may also bring a different set of experiences that can contribute to the vision. Supervisors who have been with you for a long time have probably witnessed past change attempts that failed. They may simply be biding their time to see if this all blows over before expending much effort.

If significant philosophical differences crop up, supervisors should be urged to reconsider their fit with the organization. Some may be leery but willing to change, while others may be unmoving in their lack of support for the new direction. Assessing whether these people have a future in the organization may seem harsh, but it sends the message to staff that you are completely serious about the change. It also allows supervisors who disagree with the change to find a practice setting more in keeping with their personal views, which is likely to bring them greater career satisfaction.

Step 6: Generate Short-Term Wins

By now, although your change effort will not be finished, it should be well underway. This is the time to demonstrate that you have had some short-term "wins" on the way to transforming your practice. A win is an accomplishment, not a step forward in your implementation process. In other words, creating an asthma care program is not a win, but selling it to your first patient is.

You should expect one or two small wins by the time your change effort has been underway for about six months. In fact, you should plan for your wins and decide in advance how to highlight and celebrate them before you begin to implement change.

It's hard to create a short-term win before your change effort is complete— it's a bit like trying to change the oil while leaving the engine running. You can do it, but it's messy. Short-term wins are important, though, because they motivate you to continue toward your final destination. Even small successes help reassure staff that the pain associated with change is worthwhile.

CASE EXAMPLE:
Mark Plans to Celebrate

Mark plans to celebrate the first few times his pharmacists identify and resolve drug therapy problems, since that is the thrust of the new practice. He and his staff will celebrate after pharmacists conduct the first follow-up appointments that indicate the pharmacist's intervention made a positive difference in the patient's care. They will also celebrate the first time a patient or insurer pays for the pharmacists' care.

Giving a taste of victory to your guiding coalition—which has invested time and effort to create and launch your vision—helps them see that their work was worthwhile and that their vision is sound. A short-term win also gives the coalition a sense of whether the vision needs fine tuning. Pay attention to feedback from pharmacists, physicians, and patients to be sure that what looks like a win to you is also perceived that way by others. (If it isn't, you need to evaluate your programs and perhaps make mid-course corrections.)

Showing positive results fairly quickly is a good way to convince skeptical staff that you are on the right track. This is especially valuable when the skeptics are higher up in the organization and could pull the plug if they don't see rapid signs that the new practice is a good idea. Overall, short-term wins help maintain the momentum of those involved in the change effort.

To plan for early wins, think about where your opportunities lie. Perhaps a patient has long been after you to help her stop smoking. Getting her to commit to a smoking cessation program, and seeing signs that she is sticking with it, is an early win that could help propel your patient care program forward. Or perhaps a physician has been anxious to have a pharmacist manage his patients on anticoagulants. Receiving your first referral could be a key motivator for the entire pharmacy staff.

Step 7: Consolidate Gains and Produce More Change

The change process can feel like pushing a giant boulder uphill. You peer around the edge of the rock and see the top of the mountain. You're tired and the summit looks so close, surely a little rest wouldn't hurt. From here, you can predict the rest of the story. . . . At best, loss of momentum makes reaching the top even harder. At worst, everybody is flattened under the rock as it rolls downhill. You must maintain steady progress and prevent reversal of the change everyone has worked so hard for. To do this, determine if any issues exist to prevent you from completing your change process. Scan your practice environment and try to remove barriers that remain. Admittedly, removing barriers will be more complicated in chain pharmacies or health system environments than in independent pharmacies. Ask yourself:

+ Has all training been completed?
+ Have all necessary changes in staffing and pharmacy design been accomplished?
+ Does the reward and incentive program for staff accurately reflect what you wish them to do, or are they still being rewarded for things like prescription volume or numbers of intravenous admixtures processed?
+ Do any staff remain skeptical or need more encouragement?
+ Has everything possible been done to ensure a mutually beneficial relationship with providers outside the pharmacy (if your program calls for their cooperation)?

Consolidating changes means anticipating obstacles to moving ahead and planning solutions before they are necessary. Initially, enthusiasm and adrenaline can fuel changes in the staff, but what happens when you are down one technician or a pharmacist takes maternity leave? Do the remaining staff now declare themselves "too busy" to continue the change? In Mark's case, he is the

Removing Organizational Barriers to Change

In Health Systems:

The health system environment is exactly that—a system. In this system, pharmacists provide medications and services such as drug information and pharmacokinetics. Pharmacists also seek to contribute to patient care, but they must receive cooperation, feedback, information, and referrals from other providers and departments in the system. In other words, pharmacies must capitalize on connections with other departments that have patient care responsibilities. The pharmacy manager's task is to ensure that interdependencies are strong and effective enough for pharmacists to do their jobs, but not so complicated that no one can accomplish anything without getting an okay from others. Pharmacists should be able to exchange information easily with physicians and nurses and should avoid arrangements in which they must seek permission before making patient care decisions.

In Chain Pharmacies:

Chain pharmacies are complicated environments. Each pharmacy has a front-end manager and possibly other managers who will be affected by the changes. Higher up in chain pharmacy organizations are district and regional managers who are also connected to the pharmacy. The chain may have connections to other practice groups,

continued on page 45

leader who must anticipate such hurdles. After scanning his practice to ensure that all new systems are in place—including training, staffing changes, redesign, and marketing—he's got to ask what would happen if one of those changes stalled. What if a pharmacist quits, for instance? With the help of his guiding coalition Mark should be able to identify solutions in advance, such as cross-training staff or hiring temporary help.

Step 8: Anchor New Approaches in the Culture

Suppose that your whole adult life you have been a staunch member of the Republicratic Party. A few years ago, a friend asked you to consider changing to his party—the Demopublicans. You were hesitant, but you explored the idea because he's a very close friend and a thoughtful person, and you value his opinions. Over the years, you and your

Removing Organizational Barriers to Change, continued

insurers, and suppliers, all of whom may feel ripple effects as the pharmacy changes. Managers must strive to maintain only the necessary interdependencies and should not slow the change process by keeping connections that are no longer useful. For example, a chain's policy may require that staffing changes or capital expenditures of more than $500 be reviewed by a regional manager. If so, the pharmacy manager and regional manager should determine whether this policy does more to slow down the change effort than to safeguard responsible store management.

friend have often discussed politics, and sometimes you've even voted for the Demopublicans. So finally you decide to switch political affiliations. Thanks to your friend's guidance and support, you understand the party's stance well, you believe. Then your friend moves away. He's no longer there to guide you and sometimes push you into voting for your new party. Do you think you'll continue to embrace the new political party, or will you go back to the one you belonged to before? Are you now well and truly a Demopublican, or are you still a Republicrat—albeit one with a really strong understanding of the opposition?

This analogy leads to the importance of ensuring that a patient care focus has become part of your pharmacy's culture. Culture is the shared customs, beliefs, behaviors, and social structures that make up a society. In the analogy, the Republicrats and the Demopublicans are part of a society's political culture. Your pharmacy or department is part of a business or health care culture.

At the beginning of this chapter you were asked to articulate your beliefs and values. Do they represent the cultural beliefs of patient care providers, or of some other group? Does everyone on staff believe the same thing, or are there variations in cultural beliefs?

To test whether the values, beliefs, behaviors, and structures of your new patient care culture have replaced those of your old culture, ask yourself:

+ Are all aspects of the new culture explicit to everyone in the practice?
+ Do your actions reflect your culture all the time or just some of the time?
+ Although your staff behaviors have changed, has the underlying culture changed? Are the roots of the old culture still there?

How do you change values? It's a bit like the old joke, How do you eat an elephant? One bite at a time. Changing a culture is a gradual process. Educating staff about the superiority of the new culture and cajoling them into embracing it won't work. Staff members need time to observe the new patient care focus in action and understand all its implications. Until then, talking about cultural change is probably ineffective.

Among the things you can do to promote cultural change:

+ Keep the results of your new patient care programs in front of your staff. As they see beneficial results from new programs, they will find it easier to let go and move forward, since the new culture is clearly a good one.
+ Get testimonials from patients who feel they have been well cared for with the new system. Perhaps some physicians believe the pharmacists went an extra mile for a patient. Try to gather this kind of anecdotal feedback and share it with staff to demonstrate the positive impact of new programs.
+ Continue to be supportive. Encourage two-way communication with pharmacists and technicians. Some people need to work their way through changes out loud; if they are not given the chance to vent, their transition is more difficult. Others keep their thoughts to themselves and need you to check in at times to see how they are doing. They may not volunteer their opinions unless asked, so make sure you ask them.
+ Ensure that new people you hire share your culture. Whether you realize it or not, when you hired candidates in the past you assessed whether they fit in well with the organization and what it stands for. Now you need to consciously think about the cultural fit. If you can't find the right person immediately, you may be better off filling a position later, or not at all, than filling it with someone who does not share your pharmacy's values and mission. Similarly, when promoting existing staff, be wary of allowing individuals who do not embrace the appropriate value system to rise up through the organization. Otherwise, years of effort may be undone.

It is far too soon to tell if Mark has been able to change the culture of Innovo-Medical Pharmacy. Realistically, his changes must remain in place for 3 to 5 years—during which time half his staff will turn over—before he knows for sure. If Eric, Grace, and Dee later take other jobs but Mark's new staff keep offering high-quality care (and not just customer service), then Mark can be satisfied that his change effort has been successful.

Conclusion

The change process described in this chapter takes several years. It's a sound, workable process, even though it may seem impractical to you given the pace at which health care is evolving. By the time you're only halfway toward your desired change, the marketplace will probably have changed three times. This is annoying, but to be expected. Try to keep your plans for change flexible so you can make midcourse adjustments. If the core of your new practice is genuine patient care, that will endure even if the opportunities you thought existed appear to be changing. Disease-specific educational services may or may not have a long future, but once patients have experienced true patient care, they won't want to give it up. The same is true for pharmacists who have felt the joy and pride of providing actual care to patients.

References

1. Kotter, JP. *Leading Change*. Boston, MA: Harvard Business School Press; 1996.
2. Holland RW, Nimmo CM. Transitions part 1: Beyond pharmaceutical care. *Am J Health Syst Pharm*. 1999;56:1758-64.
3. Nesbit TW, Shermock KM, Bobek MB, et al. Implementation and pharmacoeconomic analysis of a clinical staff pharmacist practice model. *Am J Health Syst Pharm*. 2001;58:784-90
4. Hepler CD, Strand LM. Opportunities and responsibilities in pharmaceutical care. *Am J Hosp Pharm*. 1990;47:533-43.
5. Anon. *Special Report: Developing Disease-Specific Pharmaceutical Care Protocols*. Washington, DC: American Pharmaceutical Association; 1995.
6. Galt KA, Narducci WA. Integrating pharmaceutical care services: the product is part of the care. *Pharmacotherapy*.1997;17:841-4.
7. Galt KA. The need to define "care" in pharmaceutical care. *Am J Pharm Ed*. 2001;64:223-33.
8. Hawthorne DL, Yurkovich NJ. Caring: the essence of health care professions. *Hum Health Care Int*. 1996;12(1):27-8.
9. Pharmacy News. Available at: http://www.pharmweb.usc.edu/apsa/pharmacynews/pharmacynews3.html. Accessed January 30, 2002.
10. Practice Environment and Quality of Worklife. Available at: http://www.aphanet.org/development/prodev.html. Accessed May 30, 2001.
11. Johnson JA, Bootman JL. Drug related morbidity and mortality: a cost of illness model. *Arch Intern Med*. 1995;155:1945-56.
12. Committee on Health Care in America, Institute of Medicine; Kohn LT, Corrigan JM, Donaldson MS, eds. *To Err Is Human: Building a Safer Health System*. Washington, DC: National Academy Press; 2000.

Chapter 3
Interdisciplinary Patient Care
June Felice Johnson

Until recently, if you were a pharmacist hoping to begin offering patient care programs, you pretty much had to make them up as you went along. Resources for helping you change to a patient-focused practice were limited in depth and breadth. Given the lack of guidance available, it is not surprising that some pharmacists have been more successful than others in moving to a new practice model.

Probably the key difference between pharmacists who have successfully implemented patient care initiatives in their practices and those who have not is this: the successful ones did not go it alone. They established solid relationships with other health care professionals who care for the same patients they do and developed clear lines of communication with other practitioners.

Pharmaceutical care cannot be practiced in a vacuum. It must be a cooperative partnership between the pharmacist, the physician, and the patient. Pharmacists who have launched workable patient care programs took the time to uncover issues important to local providers and to talk with them about targeted solutions. Those whose patient care programs have not done well typically put them into effect before finding out whether anyone was interested in the content of each program or the philosophy behind it. They picked a patient care program that was popular with other pharmacists or that piqued their interest, but they failed to discuss their choice with local providers or patients.

This chapter reflects insights from the literature as well as my personal experience in creating patient care partnerships—a concept I refer to as interdisciplinary patient care (IPC). If you use the principles of IPC, you are more likely to launch programs that meet the needs of the pharmacist, the physician, and the patient. Although this book is for managers and directors, I'm assuming that you either work on the front lines yourself at times or are closely involved in orchestrating the efforts of those who do.

IPC: A Team Approach

IPC, as applied to pharmacy practice, involves a direct and ongoing relationship between the pharmacist and one or more health care providers who work together to improve the health of a particular patient. IPC requires team members to thoroughly understand each other's unique knowledge and skills and to recognize the limits of one's own discipline in solving a patient's health problems.

Interdisciplinary Patient Care Practice Today

Following are examples of specialty practices that involve interdisciplinary, collaborative arrangements to improve patient care.

✦ **Nutrition support.** Physicians, pharmacists, dietitians, and nurses have worked together for years to address patients' nutritional problems, primarily in hospitals. Now, with the proliferation of home care services, it is becoming more common for such teams to treat outpatients as well. The American Society of Parenteral and Enteral Nutrition officially advocates an interdisciplinary role for pharmacists. To enhance their credentials, pharmacists can take an examination offered by the national Board of Pharmaceutical Specialties and become a board-certified nutrition support pharmacist.

✦ **Diabetes.** The National Certification Board for Diabetes Educators allows physicians, nurses, pharmacists, and dietitians in both community and institutional settings to earn certification as a certified diabetes educator (CDE) by completing 1000 hours of direct patient management and passing a national exam. Becoming a CDE offers several advantages. The designation is widely recognized and respected by health care providers and can be used to seek Medicare provider status.

continued on page 50

IPC can easily be confused with "collaborative practice agreements" or "practicing under protocol," which also involve cooperation among health care disciplines, but IPC is broader in its scope of responsibility. Collaborative practice typically involves a written, negotiated agreement in which both physician and pharmacist describe their responsibilities. IPC, on the other hand, involves a true give-and-take relationship in which you use independent judgment and tailor your care to the overall needs of the patient. IPC could, perhaps, be likened to a "comprehensive case management" approach in which the physician maintains overall responsibility for the patient but the pharmacist is responsible for patient education, medication adherence, and many aspects of patient monitoring.

Although collaborative practice agreements and practicing under protocol are both interdisciplinary approaches, they are also contractual arrangements. Both approaches restrict pharmacists' activities to narrowly specified services. For example, a collaborative practice agreement between a physician and pharmacist in a physician-directed, pharmacist-managed anticoagulation practice would address a narrow patient care issue—administering blood-thinning drugs, monitoring patients, and adjusting dosages—and would confine the pharmacist's responsibilities to the terms of that particular agreement. The setting for such a practice might be an outpatient clinic in a health system, the physician's office, or the pharmacy. Whatever the setting, and however the financial details are set up, a true collaborative practice always has a formal written agreement that describes who does what under which circumstances and specifies when each party should defer to the other's judgment in patient care decisions.

IPC is not a bold or even an innovative concept. If you work in a hospital, long-term care facility, or home health care agency you already interact synergistically with other disciplines to bring about positive outcomes for patients. Even so, IPC has not been broadly embraced, particularly in the community pharmacy setting.[1,2] Is there evidence to motivate the profession to move toward IPC? What are the barriers to offering IPC services and how can they be overcome? These and other questions will be explored in this chapter.

 Interdisciplinary Patient Care Practice Today, continued

✦ **Pain management.** The American Academy of Pain Management provides voluntary certification for interdisciplinary pain managers (IPM) in the areas of medicine, pharmacy, nursing, psychology, counseling, physical therapy, chiropractic, and social work. Pharmacists' involvement with pain management usually takes place in such settings as specialized pain centers, hospital-based pain management services, or hospice teams. The pharmacist's role is typically to identify or prevent drug therapy problems such as under- or overdosage, monitor the patient for adverse drug reactions and drug interactions, take part in drug selection, and recommend appropriate dosage forms and delivery systems to ensure the patient's comfort.

The Case for IPC

The need for health care disciplines to work cooperatively towards improved patient care is urgent. A recent report from the Institute of Medicine's Committee on Health Care in America noted that nearly 100,000 people die in American hospitals annually from preventable medical errors.[3] The report reviewed data on hospital admissions linked to medical errors in the states of Colorado, Utah, and New York. In extrapolating the results to national figures, researchers concluded that between 44,000 and 98,000 Americans die annually as a result of preventable medical errors, which makes them a leading cause of mortality in the United States. The total national cost of preventable medical errors was estimated at $17 billion to $29 billion in disability, health care, and lost income.

Concerns about patient safety are intensified by the growing use of innovative, expensive medications and projected increases in the number of prescriptions generated and dispensed. These trends are fueled by a progressively aging population, extended life expectancies, and increases in the number and duration of chronic health conditions. Health care payers are pressuring providers to improve patient care while seeking more value from health dollars and better outcomes from costly medications.

The sidebar on page 49 gives examples of formally sanctioned IPC arrangements to address specific health problems. Among health care systems that involve pharmacists in IPC, the Department of Veteran's Affairs (VA) stands out as a prime example because it uses both collaborative agreements, in which pharmacists and physicians establish care plans together, and interdisciplinary patient rounds. The rounds are carried out by teams of attending physicians, medical residents and students, and other health professionals. Each team manages a set number of patients. The pharmacist's role is to review the patient's medical record and medication profile to screen for drug therapy problems and suggest solutions to the team during rounds. Physicians then write orders reflecting the pharmacist's recommendations. In the VA's ambulatory care settings pharmacists have significant responsibility for patients in such areas as anticoagulation, lipid management, and diabetes management.

Outside the VA, other health care systems also have ambulatory clinics in which pharmacists are directly involved with patient management. Among the positive results that have been documented from pharmacists' efforts are an increase in office appointment compliance rates, increased medication adherence rates, increased patient satisfaction, decreased demand for physicians to spend time on routine problems, improved continuity of care, decreased rates of adverse drug events, decreased demand for emergency department or hospital care, and improved cost-to-benefit ratios for the institution.[4]

Qualities Required for Successful Teams

Anyone who wants to form a successful IPC team should be sure that the qualities listed below are represented. The degree to which each is necessary depends on the type of team you are forming, the services to be provided, your strengths and attributes, and the outcomes you are trying to achieve.

+ Coordination and administrative abilities.
+ Team facilitation skills and experience.
+ Team leadership skills and experience.
+ Previous experience as part of a team.
+ Knowledge of organizational goals and culture.
+ Technical knowledge and expertise.
+ Interpersonal and communication skills.
+ A variety of abilities and approaches.

Source: Rees F. Teamwork from Start to Finish. 10 Steps to Results. New York: Pfeiffer and Jossey-Bass Inc. 1997.

Published studies examining interdisciplinary disease state management services demonstrate the value of pharmacists in the community and ambulatory settings. In one study, pharmacists scheduled appointments every 6 to 8 weeks to educate and monitor patients with hypertension, diabetes, asthma, and elevated cholesterol, and they communicated with physicians on patients' progress. As a result, these patients' mean total health care costs declined by $293 per person compared with patients who received standard care.[5] In another study, independent community pharmacists who worked cooperatively with dietitians and physicians to manage patients with elevated cholesterol demonstrated a significant decrease in patients' total and low-density lipoprotein cholesterol. Patients reported better quality of life and increased satisfaction with the pharmacist.[6]

Project ImPACT (Improve Persistence and Compliance with Therapy), in which pharmacists spearheaded an interdisciplinary approach to lipid management, showed that the pharmacists' efforts helped improve patient outcomes.[7] Pharmacists worked closely with physicians and other health care providers to give an advanced level of care and promote patients' long-term adherence to their drug therapy. Patients who took part in Project ImPACT improved both their medication compliance and their serum lipid levels.

In the Asheville Project, pharmacists were reimbursed for providing diabetes management—with support from physicians and other health care professionals—to employees of the city of Asheville, North Carolina. [8] Physicians trained pharmacists, referred patients to them, and received feedback on each patient's status. Pharmacists met patients by appointment, took initial histories, assessed patients' needs, taught proper use of blood glucose monitors, and set goals. During monthly follow-up appointments pharmacists monitored patients' progress and reviewed blood glucose readings, which were downloaded directly from patients' monitors into pharmacists' computers. Pharmacists shared their findings with each patient's physician and the hospital diabetes education center. Compared to baseline measures at the start of the project, hemoglobin A_{1c}, lipids, quality of life, and patients' satisfaction with the pharmacist improved when rechecked 8 and 14 months later.

Despite a lack of published data, reports from many other quarters suggest that pharmacists are contributing to patient care in ever-expanding ways. For example, they are working cooperatively with physicians to provide flu shots, a much-needed activity given the low rates of immunization in high-risk populations. According to statistics collected by the Advisory Committee on Immunization Practices, only 63% of people over age 65 and only 31% of high-risk people between the ages of 18 and 64 were vaccinated for influenza virus in 1998. [9] Healthy People 2010, a public health campaign spearheaded by the U.S. Department of Health and Human Services, has established a vaccination goal of 90% for these populations. This is a goal that pharmacists can play an important part in meeting.

In one program developed in an independent pharmacy in rural eastern Iowa, pharmacists received special training, followed written protocols, and sent documentation to physicians with whom they collaborated to immunize patients at high risk for influenza.[10] To be identified as candidates for the program, patients had to be at least 60 years old or, according to pharmacy records, must have received prescriptions for chronic cardiovascular, respiratory, or metabolic conditions. From October 15 to December 6, 1996, pharmacists administered 343 doses of vaccine. No adverse events were reported or noticed in any of the patients immunized. One-third of these patients reported not having received flu shots the previous year, indicating the positive contribution of the pharmacy's program.

Models of collaborative practice agreements are now incorporated into many states' pharmacy practice acts. In 1980, in response to a physician shortage in rural areas, Washington was the first state to start collaborative drug therapy agreements or prescriptive authority protocols. Currently, several thousand physicians and pharmacists in all practice settings in Washington are involved in these agreements, according to Grant Chester, operations manager of the Washington State Board of Pharmacy (written communication, December 6, 2001). Washington's pharmacy practice act says that the practice of pharmacy includes "the initiating or modifying of drug therapy in accordance with written guidelines or protocols previously established and approved for his or her practice by a practitioner authorized to prescribe drugs." The most commonly used agreements are in the areas of emergency contraception, immunization, refills, and anticoagulation. A 14-point checklist must be submitted to the board for a specific agreement to be approved. The level of pharmacists' involvement in patient care using these models and the types of services they provide vary widely among states.[11]

Typically, collaborative practice agreements provide less opportunity for pharmacists to apply their independent judgment than newer models that are developing. For example, the Iowa Medicaid Pharmaceutical Case Management initiative, launched in October 2000, enables pharmacists to expand the use of their professional judgment and drug therapy knowledge to make independent recommendations.[12] Through this 2-year project, pharmacists and physicians receive Medicaid reimbursement for case management services they provide as a team. Participating pharmacists are trained to gather comprehensive information from Medicaid patients who, according to data from insurance claims, are at high risk for medication problems. Pharmacists schedule patients for initial assessments and use a standard form (which they send to the physician on their team) to document drug therapy problems, recommendations, and follow-up plans. When problems need immediate attention, pharmacists contact the physician by phone or fax. At the project's completion, the teams' clinical and economic successes will be compared with those of a control group of nonparticipating pharmacies.

June Felice Johnson's Experience with IPC

I have practiced IPC for almost 20 years in such areas as family practice, geriatrics, and hospice care. At Detroit Receiving Hospital and Clinics I worked with a team that included a family practice physician and a nurse practitioner. I also worked with a multidisciplinary geriatrics team in a hospital, nursing home, and clinic affiliated with Henry Ford Hospital in Detroit. In Rochester, New York, I was part of multidisciplinary teams working in hospice care, in an assisted living facility, and on a hospital unit for the frail elderly. Now I work with family physicians in their offices in the Des Moines area. My education includes a postgraduate PharmD with a concurrent gerontology traineeship and an ASHP-accredited hospital pharmacy residency. I am also a Board-Certified Pharmacotherapy Specialist and a Certified Disease Manager in Diabetes, awarded through the National Institute for Standards in Pharmacist Credentialing.

The services I offer allow physicians to focus their skills and time on diagnosis while I concentrate on preventing and resolving drug therapy problems. I have found that working directly in the physicians' office allows me to provide a much higher quality of care than if I simply filled prescriptions after patients' visits. Among my activities:

+ Reviewing patients' charts before their office appointments and collecting information about their health problems, current medications, allergies, laboratory results, diagnostic findings, and care plans.
+ Conducting assessments during patients' initial visits to determine their needs for drug therapy education.
+ Discussing suspected drug therapy problems with the physician before each patient exam.
+ Accompanying physicians into the examining room to observe the patient's history and physical exam.
+ Asking patients questions when drug therapy concerns arise and collaborating with the physician to decide how best to resolve problems.
+ Periodically reviewing charts of patients with chronic illnesses to help physicians focus on those who need the most help.
+ Educating patients about their drug therapy, using both verbal and written instructions.
+ Assembling educational packets and using videos and teaching devices to help patients understand issues and treatments related to asthma, diabetes, and osteoporosis.
+ Responding to physicians' drug information questions.
+ Providing resource materials to each of the sites where I work, including reference books, lists of key Internet sites, and access to the CD-ROM program *Clinical Pharmacology Online* to ensure that pertinent therapeutic information is available at the point of care.
+ Informing physicians about new drug therapies and explaining how they might be applied to individual patients.

continued on page 55

June Felice Johnson's Experience with IPC, continued

Here's an example of what a difference my services can make. Once, when I was questioning an elderly woman newly diagnosed with type 2 diabetes, she confided that she had not been keeping a log of her blood sugars. Although she had received a prescription for a home blood glucose meter at the last office visit and had bought it in a local pharmacy, the instructions overwhelmed her. She had given up and returned it.

I got a meter that we use for training, brought it into the exam room, and took plenty of time to demonstrate proper technique. She called the office at the end of the week to announce that she had successfully measured her blood glucose and was "…thrilled to be able to do this myself!"

Another time I was reviewing a diabetic patient's blood glucose log while I visited with him in the exam room. Despite his insistence that "everything has stayed exactly the same," I noticed a lot of variability in his blood glucose measures and questioned him closely about his insulin injection technique, method of site rotation, and type of insulin syringes. I discovered that the last time he picked up insulin syringes at the pharmacy he received ultra-short needle syringes instead of his usual ones. He was overweight and his stomach protruded visibly over his belt. Unfortunately, the stomach was this patient's preferred site for insulin injections. When I pointed out that using varying needle lengths was altering the absorption profile of his insulin, he said, "Oh, I thought my sugars were better before I got these new syringes." I switched him back to his previous syringes and his blood glucose readings improved.

Some pharmacists are surprised to hear that I am present during physical exams. I have discovered that patients are gracious about welcoming me into the exam room and often remark, "I'm glad someone is here to look at my medications" or "Two heads are better than one."

Basic Ingredients for IPC

What knowledge, skills, and attitudes must be in place for IPC to be broadly applied within a pharmaceutical care practice? First, you must genuinely care about your patients. You must also get to know them and understand their unique background. The better you are at this, the more accepting patients will be about your involvement and the more likely that your interventions will be individually tailored rather than "one size fits all."

Once I overheard a conversation between an attending physician and a staff pharmacist on a hospital unit. The pharmacist was just beginning his "pitch" to the physician about changing a patient's drug therapy when the physician said five words that stopped the pharmacist in his tracks: "Do you know my patient?" All the pharmacist had done was react to a medication order without reviewing the chart or talking to the patient, and so he was prohibited from having an impact on this physician's drug therapy choice. If physicians do not think we are primarily motivated by our personal concerns for patients' well-being, they will not be inclined to solicit our involvement.

You must have solid grounding and depth of knowledge in content disciplines that pertain to detecting and solving drug therapy problems. If your professional interpretation isn't essential—if the only information you can contribute comes from drug-interaction screening software or a pocket-sized therapeutics reference—your services will not be needed. You must make the effort to stay abreast of the medical and therapeutics literature and apply evidence-based medicine derived from the medical literature to individual patients. Your knowledge and willingness to keep learning will solidify your value to the team and make your input indispensable.

Teamwork requires a high level of interpersonal skills. You and the other team members must be able to listen actively, negotiate, act with assertiveness, communicate clearly in writing, and maintain a cooperative outlook. Being skilled in the subtleties of interpersonal communication is important when, for example, you seek clarification for why a team member did something or wants you to do something. If not handled well, seeking clarification can come across as questioning the team member's judgment.

If you want to provide IPC, you must be committed to making certain changes and to sustaining them long enough for the practice to change as a whole. You cannot assume that other providers automatically confer trust and respect to pharmacists or consider them to be pharmaceutical care experts. You must patiently and persistently spend significant time establishing and maintaining relationships with other providers.

Processes and Outcomes

The IPC approach to patient care calls for systematic processes in all aspects of care, including collecting data on outcomes. (Additional information on collecting and interpreting patient outcomes data appears in Chapter 9.) Establishing a patient-focused practice takes time. Although you are ultimately interested in knowing the results (that is, patient outcomes) of your practice, a reasonable first step in determining your practice's success may be to collect information on the processes you used to provide care. Process measures such as the number of interventions made or the percent of recommendations accepted by the team may be useful as initial markers for success. After that, you can try to monitor and assess true patient outcomes such as blood sugars, peak expiratory flow rates, and blood pressures.

IPC: Getting Started

+ **Know the needs of your patients.** What are the characteristics of the patient population you serve, such as gender, ethnicity, and age? What are the most common chronic illnesses among your patients? What is each patient's monthly prescription cost? How frequently do your patients visit the pharmacy, physician's office, emergency department, or hospital? What complaints do you hear most commonly from your patients regarding their medical care? Conducting a patient survey is a good way to get this information, which will help you focus your services.

+ **Care about your patients.** This may seem obvious, but a genuine desire to improve the quality of your patients' lives must be the foundation of IPC services. Any other primary motive will be detected by patients and providers and will cause skepticism and mistrust that undermine your efforts.

+ **Know the needs of area providers and payers.** Do local health care systems or physician groups need patient outcomes to be improved? What benchmarks for standards of care are important to health systems? Where are the problem areas? For example, do local data suggest that patients with congestive heart failure or asthma have worse outcomes than national or regional benchmarks indicate are reasonable? Do local large employers who pay for health care benefits want to ensure that the money they spend on prescription drugs is worthwhile—that is, that drugs are treating disease effectively and improving health? Is there an opportunity to get involved in public health initiatives or wellness programs? Find out who the decision-makers are in local health systems and talk with them about their organizations' health care priorities so that your IPC services address a key need.

+ **Identify pharmacists for your IPC team.** Who has the best knowledge, skills, and attitudes for the services you want to offer? See the box on page 51, "Qualities Required for Successful Teams," for a list of attributes you should seek in team members. You must also assess your team's readiness to offer a particular service. (Chapter 1 has tips on assessing the state of your practice. Chapters 5 and 6 help you prepare your staff for providing patient care.) If only some of your staff are ready, you can start by forming a core team. Then later you can train others who are interested and committed to participating.

+ **Plan visits with other health care providers on your team.** Face-to-face time is critical in discussing each member's role in an IPC service. Convenient locations may include a physician's office or a conference room at an affiliated health care institution. Conduct

continued on page 58

IPC: Getting Started, continued

meetings at the beginning of your project and periodically thereafter to define, review, and revise each person's activities, which helps avoid misunderstandings and overlapping activities.

◆ **Establish payment rates.** The rates you will charge for your service and reimbursements for each team member must be clearly established before instituting the service. Will you charge by the hour, by the patient, by the level of complexity of the visit? These questions need to be discussed and decided in advance.

◆ **Develop written policies and procedures.** Among the material to include in your guidelines are lines of authority, methods of communication (phone, fax, e-mail, regular mail), outcomes to be monitored, reimbursement rates, procedures for submitting claims, and frequency of team meetings. By putting everything in writing your providers and pharmacists will have clear, well-defined expectations.

◆ **Document your activities.** Track the ECHO outcomes (see below) decided by the team and provide corresponding documentation, such as SOAP notes (a consistent format in which you record in the patient's chart both subjective and objective data as well as your assessment of the problem and plan for addressing it) or patient care flow charts. Track both short- and long-term outcomes.

Typical outcomes that are measured in medical care are summed up by the acronym ECHO, which stands for economic, clinical, and humanistic outcomes. Economic outcomes include direct, indirect, and intangible costs associated with a particular medical intervention. Clinical outcomes are medical results such as hemoglobin A_{1c} measures. Humanistic outcomes are the effects of the disease or treatment on the patient's functional status or quality of life. Rating scales that assess physical function, social function, general health and well-being, and social satisfaction are used to assess humanistic outcomes.

You should monitor these outcomes—which can be either positive or negative—to gain a balanced view of an intervention's effects. In other words, outcomes tell you how well a team is doing its job and what results it is bringing about. Some outcomes must be measured over many months or even years, a factor to take into account when you are establishing a timeline for collecting information.

Benefits of IPC

IPC services can succeed only if they benefit patients, providers, pharmacists, and insurers. Patients may benefit by having fewer adverse drug events, improved quality of daily life, and more satisfaction with their care. Physicians and other providers may benefit from a decreased "hassle factor" in their daily work, better patient adherence to therapeutic plans, more clinic appointments kept, better monitoring and feedback on patients' status between office visits, and reassurance that patients are getting thorough education about their drug therapy.

You and your staff may benefit by enhancing patients' loyalty, developing a referral network with other trusted providers, improving career satisfaction, and contributing to cost-effective outcomes. Depending on your practice setting, you may also see a financial return on your investment in IPC. Patients are generally more willing to pay out of pocket for services if their physician has recommended them. Insurers may require a certificate of medical necessity from a physician before paying pharmacists for patient care, but establishing an IPC practice makes these certificates easier to obtain. Insurers may benefit by spending less money to cover the costs of adverse drug events, having healthier enrollees, cutting down the number of medications that enrollees need, and increasing the satisfaction of their insured clients.

Conclusion

Collaboration between providers is important in today's complex health care environment. For you and your pharmacy staff to make the most of your role in interdisciplinary patient care you must develop the appropriate knowledge, skills, and attitudes. You must also plan carefully, select capable staff, maintain positive relationships with other health care providers, and keep your mission focused on improving the lives of the patients in your care.

Characteristics of Successful IPC Teams

A few years ago I participated in a workforce demonstration project, funded by New York State, in which a multidisciplinary team cared for frail elderly patients in what was previously a general medicine hospital unit. I was a clinical pharmacy specialist in geriatrics at the time. Our interdisciplinary team was very successful at decreasing both lengths of stay and medication costs, while at the same time increasing the numbers of patients placed back into their homes instead of into a care facility.

The team—a geriatrician, social workers, nurse practitioners, a pharmacist, registered nurses, dietitians, and a quality assurance nurse—developed a close working relationship that was both rewarding and highly effective. Below I describe the ingredients of a successful collaborative effort, which I discovered during the demonstration project and in my current position in a family practice.

+ **Clarity of mission.** Everyone on the team had a clear understanding of our mission: to keep patients in hospital beds only as long as absolutely necessary, to eliminate iatrogenic morbidity in the hospital, and to get patients back to an independent level of functioning quickly. Our actions and planning were always in the best interests of the patient. **Tip:** If community and health system pharmacists maintain a focus on the *patient* rather than the *product,* they can be similarly successful.

+ **Teamwork training.** Team members spent time together in training sessions and workshops sharing expertise and enlightening each other about our roles in patient care. We discovered many areas of overlap between the disciplines, such as patient education, as well as areas where disciplines have unique responsibility. For example, pharmacists are the only ones with a high level of involvement in pharmacokinetics, drug information retrieval, drug literature analysis, therapeutics, and assessment of adverse drug reactions and interactions. The team also was trained in strategies for working together effectively and shared "bonding time" to establish relationships before the project started. **Tip:** Pharmacies involved in collaborative efforts must allocate time for interdisciplinary team members to meet and develop productive working relationships. Unlike in institutional settings where team members work down the hall, community practitioners must reach out to providers in other parts of town and work diligently to establish solid relationships.

+ **Trust.** All relationships, whether professional or personal, require trust. Our trust was initiated in team-building sessions and was solidified as we worked together toward our common mission. Although some team members may have had misgivings

continued on page 61

Characteristics of Successful IPC Teams, continued

initially, concerned that their territory would be encroached on, the opposite turned out to be true. Our informal consultations and referrals for each other's services actually grew. Through our own performance we created an increased demand and expectation for our services. **Tip:** All pharmacists must demonstrate through their unique knowledge, skills, and attitudes that they can be trusted to improve patient care safely and effectively.

✦ **Professionalism and commitment.** All team members made clear through words and actions that they would do whatever was needed to help the patient. This meant sometimes being paged during lunch or dinner breaks, staying beyond assigned shifts, coming in to check on patients over the weekend when it was not our regular shift, and getting back to each other with promised follow-up information. Everyone went the extra mile for patients. **Tip:** You should work closely with other team members to ensure that patient care issues are followed up. Being contacted at home to discuss a patient issue or coming back to the pharmacy after closing hours may be necessary. Such "above and beyond" actions speak louder than words to illustrate commitment and professionalism. Every pharmacist in the IPC team must accept responsibility for the outcomes of each patient.

✦ **Clear lines of communication.** Because the team was in the hospital most days of the week and readily accessible by pager, we had many opportunities to talk face-to-face, exchange information, and plan strategies together. We met as a team twice a week to discuss patient issues and plan for patients being discharged from the hospital. To provide a clear understanding of each member's assessments and plans, all our written notes were integrated into the progress notes section of the patient's chart. **Tip:** You must establish procedures for communicating with team members orally and in writing to avoid confusion, address issues in a timely manner, and ensure that appropriate action is taken.

✦ **Shared decision-making.** Our health care team needed a leader to reinforce the mission and ensure coordinated effort. The physician who was assigned to this role needed to know how to work with a team that shares responsibility for patient care decisions. In other words, the leader has to be comfortable with a collaborative model, in which each team member is equally empowered, and must avoid imposing an authoritarian physician-centered model of decision making. **Tip:** Make sure that all participants are empowered to make the most of their skills and talents. Seek a physician who is comfortable with the collaborative model and who appreciates the value of pharmacists' contributions to improving patients' health.

continued on page 62

Characteristics of Successful IPC Teams, continued

✦ **Knowledge and experience.** Members of our team had extensive experience and often specialized training in geriatrics or gerontology. This enabled us to share a common depth of understanding and to develop individualized care plans for our patients. **Tip:** Pharmacists becoming involved in IPC may need to enhance their skills or knowledge in a specific area so they can be as effective as possible.

✦ **Mutual respect.** We were all experienced health care providers who not only felt confidence in our skills but also respect for the unique contributions of each provider. **Tip:** Pharmacists should invest time at the beginning of any collaborative effort to openly discuss what each member "brings to the table" to strengthen the team's bonds and ensure that responsibilities are clear.

✦ **Appreciation of strengths and limitations.** Working together allowed us to tap each other's strengths for the benefit of the patient and it familiarized us with each others'— and our own—limitations. Pharmacists typically have a better understanding of pharmacokinetics than physicians, who in turn tend to have more in-depth knowledge of pathophysiology. Nurses often have better insights into the psychosocial aspects of patient care than either pharmacists or physicians. Recognizing strengths and limitations allowed us to complement each other and function as a true team. **Tip:** Pharmacists do not have to be all things to all people. Rather, they should appreciate their limitations and have a referral network of competent professionals for situations that extend beyond their capabilities.

Barriers and Solutions

Here's a list of barriers that prevent many pharmacists from providing IPC services. Suggestions for overcoming them are provided.

✢ **"I don't know where to start."** It's understandable that pharmacists without IPC experience may be reluctant to try it. You will need to provide leadership, mentoring, and staff development to support pharmacists as they develop skills and confidence. You and other managers may first need to develop your own skills and confidence before you can mentor your staff. Chapters 5 and 6 provide useful tips on mentoring and training your staff to provide patient care.

✢ **"My pharmaceutical care skills and knowledge base are not strong enough."** If pharmacists have not had a chance to apply their knowledge in a supportive, patient-centered practice, this may be a difficult barrier. Self-confidence stems from having competence in both fundamental pharmacy skills and in the pharmaceutical care process. You will need to evaluate your staff's weaknesses and identify areas for improvement (see Chapters 5 and 6). If some of your staff have the right skills, you can use them to launch your IPC service and then have them mentor other pharmacist team members over time.

✢ **"We are short staffed and barely have time to fill prescriptions, let alone add a new service."** No question, manpower shortages are affecting the ability to implement pharmaceutical care and IPC services. The best way to deal with this problem is to be sure that pharmacists' skills are used as effectively as possible. Among key strategies for making the best use of time are preparing for each patient interview so you can complete it efficiently, streamlining work flow, using automated systems, overlapping pharmacists' schedules to simultaneously handle patient care and prescriptions, and training technicians to fill new responsibilities. Making changes in the pharmacy's functioning should allow you to schedule time for planning sessions and team building, which are critical as pharmacists adapt to IPC.

✢ **"Where's the reimbursement for an IPC service?"** Although reimbursement for patient care remains a struggle, pharmacists are slowly making progress. For example, a coalition of pharmacy organizations showcased pharmacists' skills at a National Council of State Legislatures conference in 2000, educating lawmakers on the essential role pharmacists play in caring for patients. You must be vocal with state and local legislators, government planners, and insurance companies about the medication problems patients face and the ways pharmacists can help. You should

continued on page 64

Barriers and Solutions, continued

also help establish your pharmacy's reputation for providing cost-effective IPC services that decrease patient morbidity from medications and reduce the cost of managing specific medical conditions. Projects are developing around the country in which IPC and pharmacist reimbursement go hand in hand. Although payment for IPC is not yet routine, it is becoming more common and the outlook is positive. Of course, reimbursement for IPC services is complicated unless team members agree on whether they will be paid collectively or individually. Health care providers must ensure that all team members view their opportunity for reimbursement as fair and equitable.

References

1 . American College of Clinical Pharmacy. ACCP white paper: a vision of pharmacy's future roles, responsibilities, and manpower needs in the United States. *Pharmacotherapy.* 2000;20(8):991-1020.

2 . Carter BL, Helling DK. Ambulatory care pharmacy services: has the agenda changed? *Ann Pharmacother.* 2000;34:772-87.

3 . Committee on Health Care in America, Institute of Medicine; Kohn LT, Corrigan JM, Donaldson MS, eds. *To Err Is Human: Building a Safer Health System.* Washington, DC: National Academy Press; 2000.

4 . Chrischilles EA, Helling DK, Rowland CR. Clinical pharmacy services in family practice: cost benefit analysis: 1. Physician time and quality of care 2. Referrals, appointment compliance, and costs. *Drug Intel Clin Pharm.* 1984;(18):333-41, 436-41.

5 . Munroe WP, Kunz K, Dalmady-Israel C, et al. Economic evaluation of pharmacist involvement in disease management in a community pharmacy setting. *Clin Ther.* 1997:19:113-23.

6 . Shibley MCH, Pugh CB. Implementation of pharmaceutical care services for patients with hyperlipidemias by independent community pharmacy practitioners. *Ann Pharmacother.* 1997;31:713-19.

7 . Bluml BM, McKenney JM, Cziraky MJ. Pharmaceutical care services and results in Project ImPACT: Hyperlipidemia. *J Am Pharm Assoc.* 2000;40:157-65.

8 . Garrett DG. The answer to how is when: the genesis of the Asheville Project. *Pharmacy Times.* October 1998:4-31.

9 . Centers for Disease Control and Prevention. Prevention and control of influenza: recommendations of the advisory committee on influenza practices. *MMWR.* April 20, 2001;50:1-63.

10 . Ernst ME, Chalstrom CV, Currie JD, et al. Implementation of a community pharmacy-based influenza vaccination program. *J Am Pharm Assoc.* 1997;NS37:570-80.

11 . Collaborative Practice. Available at: http://www.aphanet.org/govt/govaffair.html. Accessed May 29, 2001.

12 . *Iowa Medicaid Pharmaceutical Case Management Implementation Training Manual.* Des Moines: Iowa Pharmacy Association; 2000.

Chapter 4
DEVELOPING THE INFRASTRUCTURE FOR PATIENT CARE
Richard K. Lewis, Daniel H. Albrant, & Harry P. Hagel

Although pharmaceutical care has been pharmacy's driving philosophy for a decade, pharmacotherapy does not always bring the results that patients and their health care providers desire.[1] The reasons are complex, but a fundamental one—which this chapter addresses—is that pharmaceutical care requires the right infrastructure. As early as 1990, in the article that put pharmaceutical care on the profession's radar screen, Charles Hepler and Linda Strand noted the importance of having "an organizational structure that facilitates the provision of care."[2] Ross Holland and Christine Nimmo concur, saying that the physical environment is one of three key areas to focus on when changing pharmacy practice.[3]

This chapter looks at automation and technology, staffing adjustments, policies and procedures, and related issues that lay the groundwork for effective patient care. Additional aspects of operational infrastructure are addressed in other chapters.

Infrastructure Assessment and Planning

To develop an infrastructure that supports patient care you must examine what you have in place now and think through the results you want. Rushing to change one part of the infrastructure without determining how it will affect other parts may be costly and counterproductive. For example, people sometimes embrace new technology without first analyzing its benefits in their workplace. Their enthusiasm for something new is more powerful than logic.

Identify the Ideal Practice

"Begin with the end in mind"—a concept popularized by leadership trainer Stephen Covey[4]—applies when you are planning for patient care services. Think about the activities in the box on page 67 and imagine the "ideal" practice. Create a flow diagram that shows how each process should unfold in your setting. (See the sample flow diagram in Figure 4-1.) For each step in your flow diagram, consider who will do what. When will they do it, how will they do it, and why will they do it?

You must also think about how each component of the drug use process will affect other components. For instance, if robots handle unit dose dispensing in a centralized hospital pharmacy, how will drug administration be affected on the nursing unit? Or, how will a community pharmacy's patient counseling program affect the pharmacist's availability to process prescriptions? And, as a result, how will your flow diagram be changed?

The Drug Use Process

Typical activities in the drug use process include:

✦ **Prescribing.** Deciding to use drug therapy instead of, or in accordance with, other options such as surgery, diet, and exercise.

✦ **Selecting drugs.** Choosing specific medications to treat patients in light of their conditions, characteristics, and desired outcomes.

✦ **Selecting regimens.** Determining the appropriate dosing, schedule, route of administration, and duration of therapy for each patient's needs.

✦ **Dispensing drugs.** Dispensing the selected drugs to the patient or delivering them to the patient care area.

✦ **Administering drugs.** Having patients take the drugs themselves or having drugs administered by a health care professional.

✦ **Educating patients.** Counseling patients about their medications, regimens, and diseases.

✦ **Pharmaceutical care.** Assessing drug therapy, modifying therapy, monitoring patients, and taking part in other activities (educating patients, selecting regimens) to be sure desired outcomes are met.

Source: Hutchinson RA, Lewis RK, Hatoum HT. Inconsistencies in the drug use process. _DICP Ann Pharmacother._ 1990;24:633-36.

Figure 4-1. Sample Flow Diagram for Dispensing-Related Activities

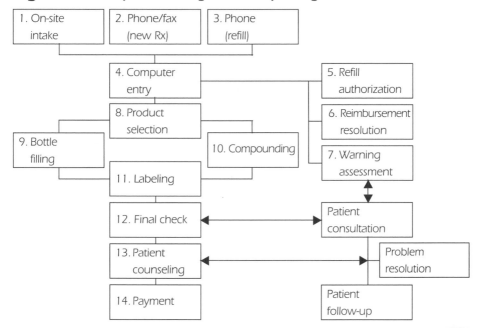

Noted Failures in the Current Drug Use Process

+ Drug-related morbidity and mortality costs are as high as $76.6 billion per year.[*]
+ 17.5% of 30 million elderly Medicare recipients are prescribed drugs that are unsafe for the age group or that duplicate therapy they are already receiving, at a cost of $20 billion in hospitalizations or $114,000 per practicing pharmacist in the U.S.[†]
+ 30% to 55% of patients deviate from their prescribed regimen.[‡]
+ 10% of all hospital admissions are related to problems in drug therapy.[§]
+ 50% of 94 discharged patients surveyed were detected to have an error in their medication regimen.[**]
+ In a study of over 1000 people with disabling injuries caused by medical treatment, 19% (the most common) of injuries were due to problems with drug therapy[††]

Sources:

*Johnson JA, Bootman JL. Drug related morbidity and mortality: a cost of illness model. Arch Intern Med. 1995;155:1949-56.

†Anon. $20 billion drug problem. PNN Pharmacotherapy Line. 1995:2 (August 14).

‡Medication Regimens: Cause of Non-compliance. Washington, DC: Office of the Inspector General, Department of Health and Human Services; June 1990:12-14.

§ Manasse HR. Medication use in an imperfect world: drug misadventuring as an issue of public policy, parts 1 & 2. Am J Hosp Pharm. 1989;46:929-44, 1141-52.

**Omori DM, Potyk RP, Kroenke K. The adverse effects of hospitalization on drug regimens. Arch Intern Med. 1991; 51:1562-4.

††Leape LL, Brennan T, Laird N, et al. The nature of adverse events in hospitalized patients: results of the Harvard Medical Practice Study II. N Engl J Med. 1991;324:377-84.

Identify Priorities

Study the flow diagram you developed to show the ideal drug use process in your setting, and think about the infrastructure you will need to support day-to-day pharmacy activities. Examples of elements you might need in your infrastructure appear in the box on page 69, top left. Probably an immediate leap to the ideal practice is beyond your financial, physical, or psychological resources, so your next step is to decide which elements are top priority and which can wait. Develop schedules for addressing each element and identify the options within each category. Because cost-effectiveness and patient safety are leading issues in health care today, any operational changes you consider should be sure to support those areas.

Automation and Technology

The new millennium has rolled in on a wave of technology that only scratches the surface of possibilities. Mind-boggling devices are in the works that have not yet hit the marketplace. Given the choices available now, and new ones entering the scene, it

Pharmacy Practice Infrastructure

Common aspects of pharmacy infrastructure include:

+ Automation.
+ Fixtures.
+ Information systems.
+ Lighting.
+ Physical layout.
+ Policies and procedures.
+ Position descriptions.
+ Scheduling.
+ Software.
+ Training.
+ Transportation and delivery.
+ Workflow.

In pharmacy, electronic prescription processing systems and electronic patient records have become common. Centralized robotic dispensing and unit-based distribution cabinets are widely used in hospitals, and automated dispensing systems are on the increase in community pharmacies. Wholesalers, large retail pharmacies, and mail order pharmacies have automated their distribution processes to achieve economies of scale as profit margins shrink. Many believe that pharmacy is not adapting to new technology fast enough, however, and the American Society of Health-System Pharmacists is working to accelerate its use.[5]

Factors Driving Automation

The primary factors driving automation in pharmacy are:

+ Consumer demand for speed, convenience, and safety.
+ Growing prescription volume.
+ Shortages of pharmacists.
+ Need to reduce medication errors.
+ Increasing role of pharmacists in patient care.

makes sense to ask these questions before adding new automation:

+ Is it needed?
+ What is the cost–benefit ratio?
+ Is it affordable?
+ What is its longevity?
+ Will it really do what I think it can do?
+ What will be needed to support it?
+ Will staff and customers accept this change?

Physicians today have powerful, expensive tools to diagnose and treat illness, but other health care technology is lagging painfully behind. Only a handful of health systems have electronic medical records (EMRs), for example, and those that have EMRs often lack important safety features, such as ways to ensure the continuity of prescription information as patients move between inpatient and outpatient status.

Putting Automation in Place

Systems that automate the dispensing and tracking of medications are tools to free pharmacists' time so they can provide patient care. When deciding how best to use automation, consider how it fits in the "ideal" drug use process you outlined earlier. Some hospitals, for example, have chosen centralized cart-fill processes in which robots use bar-code

A Sampling of Current Automation

McKessonHBOC (www.mckhboc.com)
—ROBOT-Rx: Centralized robotic cart fill system.
—AcuDose-Rx: Decentralized medication dispensing cabinet.
—AcuScan-Rx: Patient verification and drug administration tracking system.
—Drug-O-Matic, Baker Cells, and Baker Cassettes: Tablet counters for the outpatient setting.
—Autoscript III: Outpatient prescription filling (vial selection, tablet counting, and vial labeling).

AutoMed Technologies, Inc. (www.automedrx.com)
—ATC FastPak, ATC Profile, FDS: Strip packagers to support centralized cart fill or decentralized cabinets.
—QuickFill, QuickFill Plus: Tablet counters for the outpatient setting.
—FastFill, QuickScript, Opti-Fill I & II: Outpatient prescription filling (vial selection, tablet counting, and vial labeling).

Pyxis Corporation (www.pyxis.com)
—Medstation 2000 series: Decentralized medication dispensing cabinet.
—Homerus: Centralized robotic cart fill system.
—SampleStation: Dispensing cabinet for controlling samples.

Telepharmacy Solutions (www.addsinc.com)
—POC cabinets: Prepackaged medication dispensing cabinet with videoconferencing capabilities for dispensing outpatient prescriptions remotely.
—Drugsampling.com: Dispensing cabinet for controlling samples.

OmniCell (www.omnicell.com)
—OmniCell Cabinet: Decentralized medication dispensing cabinet.

Autros (www.autros.com)
—Autros Cabinet: Decentralized medication dispensing cabinet.
—Autros PDAs: Bedside medication scanner.

ScriptPro (www.scriptpro.com)
—SP200: Outpatient prescription filling (vial selection, tablet counting, vial labeling).

technology to retrieve and place into separate bins the medications for each patient. Other hospitals have moved to decentralized unit-based cabinetry, which is somewhat like having an automatic teller machine that dispenses medications rather than cash in each hospital unit. Some community pharmacies use central fill technology that allows patients' prescriptions to be prepared in a large automated facility—usually located in a different city or state—and then shipped to the local pharmacy for dispensing. Other community pharmacies have dispensing cabinets that help with selecting products, counting, filling containers, and labeling.

Automation is used in pharmacy practice for the same reasons it is used in any operation or trade: increased efficiency and reduced errors, waste, and costs. Because pharmacy automation takes over repetitive tasks, you can allot more time to other stages of the drug use process. By ensuring that processes are consistent, automated dispensing systems reduce the chance of human error, which is critical when dealing with medications. Some types of automation cut risks to personnel by keeping them away from dangerous materials such as toxic chemotherapy agents. And automation reduces waste because materials are tracked more closely, each person's accountability is clear, errors are avoided, and processes flow more efficiently.

Vendor and Product Analysis

The number of vendors offering pharmacy automation has exploded recently, making it hard to compare products' features. The sidebar on page 70 lists current vendors and their offerings. It is not comprehensive, however, and may become outdated quickly as new technology is introduced. An excellent resource to help pharmacists stay abreast of new technology developments is a Web site hosted by the Neuenschwander Company, a consulting business focusing on pharmacy automation. Go to http://www.pharmacyautomation.com.

Developing the RFP or RFI

Before you can select a vendor, you need to develop a list of criteria the automation is expected to meet. For example, you may know that you want the automated system to track inventory, reconcile purchasing invoices with payments and shipments, and interface with the pharmacy software. An effective approach for ensuring that vendors provide the detailed information you want—especially if you have a deep understanding of pharmacy automation—is to use a Request for Proposal (RFP) or a Request for Information (RFI).

An RFP is a detailed document you develop and send to potential vendors asking them for a formal proposal describing their products and services. An RFI is, in simple terms, an open-ended RFP that allows potential vendors to explain what they think the buyer needs to know. RFIs are less specific than RFPs and are particularly helpful when buyers are unsure what they want or need. Because it is so hard for buyers to

keep up with all the new technology emerging today, RFIs are becoming more popular. Doing an RFP would be overwhelming if, for example, you don't know whether
you prefer centralized cart-fill automation or decentralized unit-based cabinets. The
RFI process can help identify the advantages and disadvantages of both.

If you're doing an RFP, you'll find it's a challenge to put all the details and possibilities of an automation project in writing. The flow diagrams you developed to
illustrate your ideal practice (see page 66) should help you think carefully about your
needs. In the RFP it's important to include all the features you're seeking, because the
RFP will likely serve as the basis for the contract, the implementation timeline, and
the overall relationship with the vendor. Include all interested parties in the RFP development process, including owners and outside contractors. Make sure that engineering personnel evaluate electrical needs, compressed air requirements, and other
technical specifications. Construct a timeline for the project and share it with the vendors you are considering (see Figure 4–2).

Whenever possible, give potential vendors a checklist of functions and features
you are seeking in your new automation.
(See the sample checklist in Figure 4-3.)
When including "yes or no" questions,
phrase them so the desired answer is always "yes" or always "no." This lets you
quickly scan the responses to identify areas that may be a problem for the vendor.

Figure 4-2. Example of a Buyer's
Anticipated Project Timeline

✓ Jan 30 - RFPs sent to selected vendors.
✓ March 1 - Response to RFP due. (*Rushing
  the vendor for an RFP response may not
  be in the buyer's best interest. Give the
  vendor reasonable time to respond
  accurately.*)
✓ April 20 - Successful bidder notified.
✓ April 22 - Purchase order for project
  issued.
✓ May 1 - Initial project meeting held with
  selected vendor.
✓ May 30 - Implementation process begins.
✓ October 1 - Site goes live.

Common Elements of Vendor Proposals

A typical Request for Proposal asks
vendors to include the following
sections:

✦ Executive Summary that describes
  the approach the vendor will use
  to implement the project and the
  expected costs.
✦ Corporate information, including
  financial details.
✦ List of current customers and
  contact information.
✦ Functions the automation must
  carry out and features it
  should have.
✦ List of proposed implementation team
  members and their qualifications.
✦ Proposed implementation
  schedule.
✦ Costs and payment details.
✦ Terms and conditions.

Figure 4-3. Checklist of Desired Functionality and Features

CA = Currently available and installed with current customers
UD = Under development (enter expected availability date)
Cust = Customization required (attach time and cost details)
N/A = Not available

Feature/functionality	CA	UD	Cust	N/A
		mm/dd/yy		
Interface with pharmacy software system (host to automation)				
Interface with pharmacy software system (automation to host)				
Ability to fill all dosage forms:	——	——	——	——
Tablets				
Capsules				
Liquids				
Creams/Ointments				
Inhalers				

Maximum number of medications stored: _____

Floor space required for automated device:_____ Sq. Ft.

Floor space required for automated device and support activities: _____ Sq. Ft.

Ceiling height required: _____

Is compressed air necessary? Y   N

If yes, please list specifications (i.e., PSI, "clean" air, etc.)

Variables to Consider

When you are developing an RFP or evaluating potential suppliers' responses, you need to consider many different elements. The following advice, though far from comprehensive, gives you key pointers.

Price and Leasing or Purchasing

Because the cost of buying or leasing equipment is such a major factor, you must identify all costs, not just the "sticker price." Buyers are often surprised, for example, when they discover the cost of interfacing the automation with the pharmacy's or hospital's computer system. Shake out all costs in advance, not after you've signed a contract or installed your equipment. Examples of ancillary costs to account for are:

- Installation.
- Interfaces with the current computer system.
- Software.

+ Supplementary equipment.
+ Supplies.
+ User training.
+ Maintenance.

After you've tallied the full cost of getting new equipment up and running, compare it with the cost of doing things the current way. You may find that automation will cut costs by reducing the staff you need, or it may increase your revenue because you can handle a bigger prescription volume. A payback analysis (see box on page 75) can be particularly helpful because it allows you to calculate how long it will take for the automation to pay for itself.

Many vendors offer lease programs that allow you to spread the cost of automation over time and avoid an up-front capital expenditure. Through a payback analysis you can determine whether it makes more sense to make a capital expenditure and lose that money's earning power or to lease the equipment and pay the related fees.

Vendor Support
Check to be sure that the vendor provides good customer support. You need to know how and when vendors will respond to problems with the automation. What is the vendor's approach to providing support? How soon after you call for help will the vendor respond? What does the vendor charge for support? Many vendors offer phone support within 1 hour and on-site support within 24 hours if the problem cannot be resolved by phone within 6 hours. The vendor's support is likely to come with a fee. Negotiate the support costs early on to avoid problems later.

Interfaces
When automation is being installed or maintained, some of the biggest headaches have to do with interfaces between equipment or systems. What it usually boils down to is that you are dealing with two vendors, neither of whom wants to incur additional costs or expend extra effort. If an interface problem occurs, each vendor will be inclined to point a finger at the other one.

Wording Tip

Be cautious about using the words "required" or "must" in the RFP. Instead, use vocabulary that is less absolute, such as "desired" or "optimal." If vendors think a specific feature is essential or a timeline is immovable, they may decide not to respond—and you may miss out on an otherwise excellent supplier. Alternatively, some vendors may stretch the truth because they're afraid they won't be considered for the project if they admit they can't offer that exact feature or schedule.

Simple Payback Analysis

This example evaluates direct costs only. In your payback analysis you may want to include the cost of financing or the opportunity costs of an up-front purchase (for example, the cost of not having that money in an interest-bearing account).

+ **Cost of automation:** $300,000
+ **Technician salary** (with benefits): $35,000
+ **Payback** (assuming a reduction of two full-time techs): $300K ÷ $70K = 4.3 years

Rest assured that vendors who want to sell you their products will say interfacing is simple and "no problem." Get it in writing, with all the details spelled out. And be sure to find out what your current computer vendor charges to work on an interface with new automation. Ask how much advance notice your computer vendor needs to assist with an interface and how many days or weeks they expect the task to take.

Calibration

Automated equipment that stores drug products in canisters typically has settings that must be adjusted according to the product's size and shape. You should find out whether your staff will be able to calibrate the canisters themselves. If not, what will it cost to send canisters to the vendor for calibration, and how long will it take?

Ancillary Expenses

Equipment costs do not necessarily stop with the purchase or leasing price. Some automation requires specific types of labels, paper, vials, or bar-coded packaging that must be placed over unit-dose medications, for example. You will need to evaluate the costs and availability of these items. You don't want your operation to come to a halt simply because the supply of a certain kind of container has dried up.

Adaptability

Plan ahead to be sure the automation can accommodate potential changes in workload. If you are expecting a large increase in the volume of prescriptions, will the automation be able to increase capacity accordingly? What additional costs will be associated with expanding the equipment's capacity?

Implementation Issues

Automation is not going to solve all your problems and create rocket-fast efficiency. Expect a learning curve and bumps in the road before things function smoothly. Pharmacy automation currently on the market does not automate the entire drug use process or even the entire dispensing process. You may find that automation eliminates the prescription-filling bottleneck in your operation but that a new bottleneck materializes in the prescription checking or counseling process.

Quality Control

No matter which automated system you install, your responsibility to maintain quality control doesn't change. It's critical to provide quality control mechanisms to ensure that prescriptions are filled and labeled accurately and that drug inventory is stored and secured appropriately. Quality control procedures should be spelled out in detail so they are always performed consistently, and they should be tested regularly. Quality control issues to consider before you put automated systems into use include:

+ **Stocking mechanisms.** Be sure you have procedures in place so that no errors occur when machines or machine cassettes are stocked.
+ **Documentation.** Procedures for labeling, packaging, and filling must be handled in a way that ensures patient safety and that meets all laws and regulations.
+ **Garbage in Garbage out.** GIGO is a common acronym that computer specialists use to describe what happens when inappropriate information is entered into a computer. If the incorrect drug is entered into the pharmacy software, the automation is going to give you what you asked for: the wrong drug. Quality checks must be in place to catch human error. And more importantly, procedures must be developed to ensure that mistakes do not occur in the first place.

Legal and Regulatory Issues

Pharmacy is a tightly regulated profession. Not only is it governed by strict laws, but it adheres to standards developed by professional associations and accrediting bodies such as the Joint Commission on Accreditation of Healthcare Organizations and the National Committee for Quality Assurance. These regulations and standards often deal with the control and security of pharmaceutical products, but their ultimate goal is to ensure public safety.

Key Legal and Regulatory Issues Regarding Automation

The following issues may vary from state to state:

+ Whether pharmacists are required to verify doses dispensed from automated devices.
+ Who is authorized to stock automated devices with medications.
+ What requirements govern controlled substance counts.
+ What requirements govern the security of legend drugs and controlled substances.
+ Whether electronic signatures are valid.

Until recently, pharmacy's regulatory bodies focused primarily on drug distribution. About 90% of regulators' efforts went into the part of the drug use process that causes less than 10% of patients' drug-related problems. Today, a growing number of regulations are being enacted that recognize the role pharmacists play in activities other than drug distribution. For example, long-term care has had drug use review requirements in place for years. The Omnibus Budget Reconciliation Act of 1990 (OBRA '90) made it mandatory for pharmacists to counsel Medicaid patients about their medications and to perform prospective drug use review. Soon after OBRA '90 went into effect, states enacted regulations that extended the provisions to all patients. Now many state pharmacy practice acts include provisions that allow pharmacists to engage in collaborative care arrangements with physicians and to prescribe or adjust pharmacotherapy under approved protocols.

Enacting regulations regarding automated dispensing devices is tough because not all systems operate the same way or focus on the same part of the distribution process. Even so, many states have added language to their pharmacy practice acts that addresses automation. See the sidebar on page 76 for a summary of regulatory issues.

Justifying the Dollars

New automation is usually a capital expenditure that must be justified to the person (or people) responsible for the organization's finances. In a community pharmacy this may be the owner, the manager, or even stockholders. In a health system it may be a chief financial officer or, more than likely, a board of directors. To convince the "holder of the funds" that a new expenditure has merit you must delineate the features and benefits clearly, in terms consistent with the organization's goals. For more on this topic refer to Chapter 7, which covers business plan development.

Although the main purposes of automation are typically to increase efficiency and reduce errors, waste, and costs, these are only words unless your success in achieving such goals is supported by actual or projected data you can use to calculate a return on investment.

Efficiency

Increasing efficiency can be defined quite simply as doing more with less without reducing quality—and perhaps even improving quality. Unfortunately, the "less" is often translated to staffing hours. Ask yourself, Will the pharmacy actually be able to process orders and fill prescriptions faster and more accurately with reduced numbers of staff? To quantify your savings, determine the specific tasks that automation will either augment or eliminate. Then estimate the amount of staff time currently required to complete each task.

One of the many ways to measure staff time spent completing tasks was described by Nickman, et al.[6] To get a sense of their methodology, imagine that a new dispensing robot will make it unnecessary for technicians to fill medication carts and will simultaneously reduce the need for pharmacists to check individual patient bins. Work sampling indicates that approximately 2 hours of technician time and 1 hour of pharmacist time will be saved every day. If you extrapolate these findings you realize it's possible to save 730 technician hours and 365 pharmacist hours annually. Assuming an average hourly salary and benefit package of $10 per hour for technicians and $40 per hour for pharmacists, this translates to nearly $28,000 annually.

Of course it is difficult to reduce full-time employees' schedules by only 1 or 2 hours per day, but you may find ways to reduce staffing levels at various times of the day to decrease payroll expenses. You might even eliminate an entire position through attrition, since many pharmacies are having trouble recruiting pharmacists and technicians these days. However, most pharmacy managers don't like that solution and would prefer to reallocate the hours saved to activities that could potentially lower costs in other areas, such as formulary management, patient monitoring, and patient compliance.

The pharmacy literature suggests that, on average, $16 can be saved in medication and other care-related costs for every dollar spent on a pharmacist engaged in patient care.[7] This statistic alone is a strong argument for ensuring that pharmacists provide effective patient care. If you give technicians the technical tasks currently performed by pharmacists, a total of 3 hours per day is made available for pharmacists to provide patient care. Using a very conservative cost–benefit ratio of 1 to 4, the savings amount to nearly $180,000 annually.

Reducing Errors

A recent survey conducted by the American Society of Health-System Pharmacists suggests that more than 60% of patients admitted to hospitals in the United States are concerned that they might receive the wrong medication.[8] And actual reports of this happening in hospital and community pharmacy settings have gotten prominent coverage in the news. When a pharmacy or health system finds itself involved in such a disaster, patients' loyalty and trust is seriously damaged. Health care's competitive nature makes customer satisfaction a high priority for owners, managers, and administrators.

The value of satisfaction and loyalty is hard to put in monetary terms, but if reducing errors is one way to keep customers, then surely automation is a worthwhile step. An automated dispensing process with virtually 100% accuracy is a reassuring investment for anyone responsible for reducing legal exposure, avoiding bad publicity, and building customer volume.

Reducing Waste, Increasing Payments

Automation accelerates inventory turnover so fewer products expire before they are used, which decreases inventory costs. Automation also improves overall cash flow by capturing usage patterns. Because computerized systems detail when medications are used, who administers them, and who receives them, third-party reimbursement rates go up and the number of charges denied because of poor record-keeping at the health care facility drops. Automation makes insurance claims far easier to reconcile. As a result, you capture more dollars directly, and indirectly you gain investment income from those same dollars.

Reducing Costs

As noted in the section on efficiency, automation lets you reallocate pharmacists' time to patient care activities and reduce both medication-related costs and expenditures for medical services. One example, published by Mutnick, et al.,[9] describes how to estimate the cost of undesirable patient outcomes that might have occurred had they not been averted by pharmacists' interventions.

Costs can also be contained indirectly by using an automated telephone reminder system to improve patient compliance, which has the potential to reduce unnecessary physician office visits and hospitalizations. Now that health systems are expanding to include hospitals, community pharmacies, and even health plans, they have a greater stake in seeing that patients adhere to their medication regimens.

For the last several decades, pharmacy benefit companies have saved money by using more formulary products and generic medications. Computerized prescribing has the potential to cut costs because it provides immediate feedback to help physicians select the proper medication and adhere to the formulary. Knowing your formulary adherence rate and your usage levels of generic medications, as well as your potential for improving these areas, can help you quantify cost savings. Computerized prescribing systems also alert you to potentially incorrect doses and provide access to critical drug information, which increases patient safety and reduces the risk of adverse events.

Convincing Decision-Makers

How you justify the expense of new technology will, of course, depend on your circumstances. Health care today is strained by rising costs and beleaguered by concerns about quality, which means that improved patient care must be balanced by financial reality. When you gather information through RFPs or RIFs, consider how the automation will help you reach both your departmental goals and those of your organization. Doing your homework and being prepared to substantiate your projections will put you in a better position to convince those who hold the purse strings that money for automation and technology will be well spent.

In Summary: Benefits of Currently Available Pharmacy Automation

+ **Accountability.** Computerization and bar coding allow nearly all drugs dispensed to be tracked by the patient, physician, nurse, or pharmacist. This is especially useful for controlled substances, because you are able to know the exact quantity you have in your inventory at all times. Without this feature, the only information typically available at the time a drug is administered is the dose and quantity prescribed.

+ **Error prevention.** The sophisticated tracking ability of bar coding and computerization, the reduced need for human oversight, and the pharmacy's ability to control drugs in operating rooms, emergency departments, and other areas cuts the potential for error.

+ **Improved efficiency.** Automation makes nearly all parts of the drug distribution process more efficient. The pharmacy invests less time because many manual processes are eliminated and there are fewer filling errors to correct. Nurses in both inpatient and long-term care settings invest less time because they no longer must count narcotics manually or deal with keys to lock-boxes that hold controlled substances. And they have fewer missing doses to account for, which saves time as well.

+ **Accessibility with control.** Many automated devices allow medications to be obtained as needed, which eliminates emergency deliveries from the pharmacy, particularly in long-term care settings, where access can be controlled by off-site computers.

+ **Charge capture.** Because automated devices can track and correlate inventory with each patient who receives medications, they improve billing processes and patient data collection.

Using Pharmacy Technicians

In pharmacies that cannot justify the capital expense of automation, pharmacy technicians are helpful in freeing pharmacists from drug distribution tasks. Two important questions to answer are:

+ Which tasks can be delegated to technicians?
+ What systems must be in place to ensure patient safety?

To safely expand technicians' responsibilities you must change their old habits, implement appropriate training programs, and establish methods to assess their competency.

Typical Duties in Pharmacy Operations

Medication Distribution

+ Procuring and maintaining the drug inventory.
+ Receiving the prescription order or refill request.
+ Obtaining or updating the patient's information.
+ Reviewing the prescription for completeness.
+ Clarifying the prescription order, if necessary, for processing.
+ Entering the prescription order into the computer.
+ Performing drug use review and evaluating any computer-generated warnings that come up.
+ Selecting the product and retrieving it from the shelf.
+ If necessary, compounding the product or formulation.
+ Preparing the medication for dispensing.
+ Labeling the medication.
+ Dispensing the medication to the patient.

Administrative and Operational

Processing charges and resolving problems such as payment denials.
Preparing reports and records.
Doing general housekeeping and maintenance.
Supervising and training new staff.
Handling complaints and problems.
Answering the telephone.
Delivering medications and supplies.

Changing Old Habits

First you must evaluate each activity in the pharmacy and determine whether it needs to be performed by pharmacists or technicians. The primary goal is to minimize the amount of time pharmacists spend in product-related activities. Although pharmacists are ultimately responsible for this aspect of pharmacy practice, their hands-on efforts can often be reduced to final checks of filled prescriptions. Countless other tasks related to drug distribution and pharmacy operations can be delegated to technicians so pharmacists are free to interact with patients.

The sequence of steps in the drug distribution process typically begins with procuring medications and maintaining the drug inventory and ends with giving the patient a prescription drug that has been dispensed and labeled accurately. (See sidebar at left.)

Work Activity Analysis

This section outlines a step-by-step process for analyzing work activities to determine staffing implications. (We originally described this process in Chapter 7 of the book *A Practical Guide to Pharmaceutical Care*.[10]) The goal of this analysis is to reduce pharmacists' involvement in distribution and administrative tasks. First you list the distribution and administrative tasks in your pharmacy, as shown in the sidebar at left.

Next you determine the percentage of time or "relative contribution" that pharmacists and technicians spend on each activity. If you think of the overall time allocated to each task as 100%, what por-

Table 4-1. Sample Pharmacy Staff Contribution Worksheet

	Current Relative Contribution		Desired Relative Contribution	
	RPh	Tech	RPh	Tech
Medication Distribution Activities				
1. Procure/maintain drug inventory	30%	70%	5%	95%
2. Receive prescription/refill request	65%	35%	10%	90%
3. Obtain refill authorization	80%	20%	20%	80%
4. Obtain/update patient information	40%	60%	20%	80%
5. Review prescription for completeness	95%	5%	50%	50%
6. Clarify Rx/order for processing	95%	5%	50%	50%
7. Enter Rx/order into computer	95%	5%	50%	50%
8. Assess DUR warning	100%	0%	75%	25%
9. Select/retrieve product from shelf	65%	35%	5%	95%
10. Compound product/formulation	65%	35%	5%	95%
11. Prepare medication for dispensing	25%	75%	5%	95%
12. Label medication	25%	75%	5%	95%
13. Dispense medication to patient	90%	10%	50%	50%
Administrative/Operational Activities				
14. Process reimbursements/charges	50%	50%	5%	95%
15. Prepare reports/records	50%	50%	10%	90%
16. General housekeeping/maintenance	50%	50%	5%	95%
17. Supervise/train new staff	75%	25%	25%	75%
18. Handle complaints/problems	75%	25%	25%	75%
19. Answer the telephone	50%	50%	10%	90%
20. Deliver medications/supplies	25%	75%	5%	95%
TOTAL RELATIVE CONTRIBUTIONS	**1245%**	**755%**	**435%**	**1565%**
NET RELATIVE CONTRIBUTIONS	**62%**	**38%**	**22%**	**78%**

tion of that time is handled by pharmacists and what portion by technicians? For the task of receiving new prescription orders and refill requests, for example, what percentage of time does a pharmacist spend versus a technician?

After that, decide which activities absolutely must be performed by pharmacists because of the knowledge and training required or because of laws and regulations. Objectivity is important when evaluating tasks: do not be swayed by the traditional dispensing paradigm in most pharmacies. In staff meetings, discuss each task openly and give everyone the opportunity to voice their opinions. Evaluating tasks requires teamwork and a genuine desire to challenge old habits for the good of patients and the pharmacy. Afterwards, address any real or perceived barriers to assuming new roles and responsibilities (see Chapters 2 and 5).

Then, as the example in Table 4-1 shows, you add up the relative contributions of pharmacists and of technicians to determine the total relative contributions. Divide those totals by the total number of activities. The total relative contributions of the pharmacists in Table 4-1 is 1245%. When you divide that figure by 20 (the total number of activities) the net relative contribution is 62%.

Calculating Staffing Adjustments

Estimate the actual number of hours that can be made available for patient care by changing the percentage of time pharmacists contribute to each task. To do this, first determine the total number of pharmacist staffing hours scheduled each week. Second, have pharmacists estimate the average percentage of total daily work time they devote to distribution activities and to administrative/operational tasks. Each pharmacist must ask herself or himself "How much time do I spend on distribution?" and "How much time do I spend on administration and operations?"

Table 4-2, which shows data for the sample pharmacy, is a guide for assembling the necessary information and performing the calculations. Pharmacists at the sample pharmacy estimated that they spend approximately 60% of their time on distribution-related tasks and 30% on administrative/operational tasks. (The remaining 10% of their time is for breaks and miscellaneous activities.) If pharmacists work a total of 200 hours per week at the sample pharmacy, this means 180 of those hours are devoted to distribution and administrative functions.

Table 4-2. Sample Pharmacy Staffing Adjustment

CURRENT STAFFING HOURS	
Pharmacist Hours Scheduled Per Week	200 Hours
Current Distribution Staff Hours	
Average Percent of Overall Time	60%
Estimated Hours	120 Hours
Current Administrative/Operational Staff Hours	
Average Percent of Overall Time	30%
Estimated Hours	60 Hours
TOTAL	**180 Hours**
NON-PATIENT CARE HOURS	
Current Net Relative Contributions (Table 4-1) 62%	
Desired Net Relative Contributions (Table 4-1) 22%	
Net Decrease in Contribution to Non-patient Care	**65%**
Potential Hours Made Available for Patient Care	**117 Hours**

To estimate the number of hours potentially available for pharmacists to provide patient care, subtract the desired net relative contribution from the current net relative contribution. In the sample, 62% minus 22% is 40%. Then divide 40% by the current net relative contribution (62%) to arrive at the net decrease in contribution to nonpatient care. In the sample, the net decrease is 65%, which translates to 117 hours per week. In other words, 117 hours should now be available for pharmacists to provide patient care.

Making Staffing Adjustments

The work activity analysis is a powerful tool for developing consensus and getting your pharmacy team's commitment to changing the way work is carried out. But estimating the potential pharmacist hours for patient care is only an exercise unless you actually reassign tasks to technicians and carry out strategies to change workflow.

Although it's possible to make sweeping changes and address all work activities at once, usually it's better to focus first on a few tasks technicians are already performing that have the greatest potential to free pharmacists' time. This keeps down the amount of technician training necessary and still frees up pharmacists for patient care.

For example, if during busy periods technicians help pharmacists enter prescription orders into the computer, you could assign primary responsibility for that task to technicians. Computer entry often takes a great deal of pharmacists' time, which now can be redirected to patient care. Because the technicians are already capable of computer entry, reassignment only requires pharmacists and technicians to agree to the new responsibilities. If, however, some technicians are uncomfortable with the new responsibilities or the pharmacists feel additional training is advisable, you can develop a schedule of training to complete within a specified period of time. Then you can establish an implementation timeline and select training methods for each additional task you plan to reallocate from pharmacists to technicians.

Assigning new tasks to technicians nearly always requires you to schedule additional technician hours during the workday. It's important to recognize this early in the process and reassure technicians that they will not be asked to assume a greater work load without considering their current time constraints. You can assign tasks that do not require special technician skills to clerical staff or hire less skilled staff at a lower salary.

To figure out when to schedule additional technicians, identify the time of day when the pharmacist or technician currently performs the task being delegated. The trickle-down effect complicates the process but can be overcome with careful planning. For example, if a technician spends afternoons handling drug returns, placing new orders, or handling other inventory functions and now is expected to enter prescription orders into the computer, another staff person will have to take over the inventory-related functions. The best answer is to add clerical staff during the time of day the inventory tasks need to be completed.

Preparing Technicians for New Roles

Chapter 5's strategies for motivating staff to provide patient care and Chapter 6's advice about education and training apply to technicians, not just pharmacists. The only variable is the tasks technicians are trained for. Fortunately, a growing number of resources are available to help technicians acquire new skills. Furthermore, mechanisms are now in place to verify that technicians have at least a baseline level of knowledge.

The Pharmacy Technician Certification Board (PTCB), formed in 1995 by several national and state pharmacy organizations, has achieved tremendous success. From 1995 to early 2002 more than 104,000 pharmacy technicians in the United States were certified by the Board, suggesting a growing awareness of the value technicians bring to the profession. PTCB provides a nationally recognized examination to assess candidates' knowledge and offers training materials and sample job descriptions for technicians practicing in all settings. For complete information, visit the PTCB Web site at http://www.ptcb.org.

Policy and Procedure Manuals

Philosophies tend to conflict regarding the role of policies and procedures in pharmacies. One camp perceives them as constraints that inhibit professional problem-solving and reduce the staff's ability to address issues creatively. Another considers policies and procedures essential to make sure tasks are performed consistently and to offer guidance about training, education, and disciplinary actions. Whatever your philosophy, when you move into a new arena like patient care you need some type of written document outlining expectations and processes. The document's level of detail and comprehensiveness depends on the complexity of your operation and the degree of overlap in job responsibilities.

The most common problem with policy and procedure manuals is their tendency to get outdated quickly. Sometimes they contain policies generated in reaction to a specific, short-term problem and thus they lack insight into system issues that produced the problem in the first place. Often they don't have a useful index or table of contents, so users can't find key material. Manuals are relegated to a shelf until a controversy develops or you need to demonstrate their existence for legal, regulatory, or accreditation purposes.

The most useful question you can ask yourself when updating or creating a manual is, "If I were a new employee, how would I determine what is expected of me, the standards I will be held accountable for, and the tasks I must carry out?"

Before You Start Writing

A common flaw in manuals is the authors' failure to consider the difference between a policy, a procedure, and a task (see box below). A policy is meant to set the ground rules by which a group interacts and makes decisions over time. Policy statements should be forward-looking and broad enough to encompass a changing practice picture. A procedure should clearly describe the steps required to achieve a reproducible result from a given task. Procedures should be written when a task, such as preparing a highly toxic medication, needs to be completed the same way each time.

Policies and procedures are related, but different. You can have standalone policies; policy statements with associated procedures (such as policy on a specific patient service and a procedure for enacting the policy); or standalone procedures (such as the procedure for compounding a specialty product).

Before writing a policy or procedure, stop and ask why you're creating the document. What is the material's purpose? Make it a rule to have a purpose statement in all policies. This creates the focus necessary to write a clean, clear document and it allows future managers and employees to assess whether the policy has outlived its usefulness. Also, ask yourself if the problem you are about to address is an isolated incident, perhaps involving a specific physician or employee. If it is, deal with the person separately rather than creating a policy or procedure.

If a policy or procedure will be in use for a limited time, place an expiration date on top. Once that date has passed, review the material to see if the issue has been resolved or the date needs to be extended. A manufacturer or wholesaler outage of a popular medication is an example of an issue that could be dealt with by a limited-time policy.

Assembling the Manual

Most policy and procedure manuals have three major sections: human resources management, distribution and clinical operations, and continuous quality improvement. Typically, each section has several subsections.

 Key Definitions

+ **Policy:** A definite course of action used to define present and future decisions.
+ **Procedure:** A series of steps followed in a prescribed order.
+ **Task:** An assigned piece of work.

Human Resources Management

The number of legal and performance-related issues that arise can cause pharmacy managers great distress, no matter what size the organization. If your pharmacy does not have access to a human resources department, it's worthwhile to get help from human resources consultants, which you can find through your local Chamber of Commerce, Rotarians, or Small Business Administration office. The Internet also has listings of human resource professionals, associations, and informational material.

Orientation

The orientation portion should be tailored to each type of employee on staff. You can have one broad section for technicians involved primarily in dispensing, but a technician who mainly does purchasing needs a totally different section. The more specialized the personnel, the more specialized the orientation section. If new equipment is installed or the staff reporting structure is changed significantly, the orientation section needs to be updated.

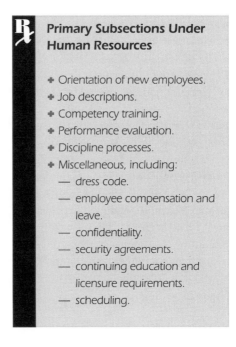

Primary Subsections Under Human Resources

+ Orientation of new employees.
+ Job descriptions.
+ Competency training.
+ Performance evaluation.
+ Discipline processes.
+ Miscellaneous, including:
  — dress code.
  — employee compensation and leave.
  — confidentiality.
  — security agreements.
  — continuing education and licensure requirements.
  — scheduling.

Include a checklist in the orientation section to ensure that each employee receives the same information in the same way and that nothing important is overlooked.

Job Descriptions

Community pharmacies and other small businesses often fail to use job descriptions because everyone just "does what needs to be done." But job descriptions are important because they clearly describe how the employee contributes to the overall operation, lend stability to the organization, and facilitate employee advancement.

Job descriptions are also cost-effective because they avoid lost productivity and wasted training time. Here's an example. In the average community pharmacy, small community hospital, or nursing home, everyone has probably worked together for years and has determined his or her place in the pecking order. When there is a vacancy, the manager struggles to determine what qualities and experience the new person should have and defaults to seeking a person who seems similar to the one who left. Because the manager doesn't truly understand the vacant job, he or she may hire someone totally unsuitable who has trouble learning the ropes and unknowingly aggravates the staff. The new employee gets frustrated and leaves for another job.

Using job descriptions to inform potential employees about their responsibilities allows them to decide if they are a good fit. Otherwise, employees are left with an oral description of expectations, which can change markedly over time. Job descriptions allow employees to understand other positions and groom themselves for promotions.

Performance Evaluations

Once the job has been described, it's a straightforward process to evaluate employees and to take disciplinary steps if they become necessary. Forms used for performance evaluations typically include a rating scale with explanations of what each number represents (for example, 1 = not meeting job expectations and 5 = exceeds all job expectations). According to human resource professionals and experienced managers, most employees fall in the mid-range: "meets all job expectations."

Good performance evaluation forms include a section where you describe the employee's strengths and weaknesses as well as a section for stating goals for the coming year and defining two or more measurable achievements you expect.

℞ What to Include in Job Descriptions

To be useful, job descriptions should be specific to the job classification, such as assistant director. They should also include the following information:

+ Baseline knowledge and experience requirements.
+ Required special skills (e.g., word processing, budget management).
+ Normal duties and expectations.
+ Work hours (both daily and weekly).
+ Reporting structure (who they manage and who they are managed by).
+ Pay grade or salary.
+ Continuing education requirements to maintain the position.

Most managers prefer a participatory evaluation process in which employees take the form and rank themselves in advance. When employees rate themselves above the mid-range, ask for examples of work that demonstrate this score. By the same token, if you rate employees lower than the mid-range score, give concrete examples of how they failed to meet expectations. Describe the coaching and assistance they will receive and note the specific improvements that are needed. This paperwork not only helps employees understand exactly how they must improve, but it also serves as key documentation if poor performance leads to the discipline process.

You should explain the performance evaluation process and philosophy well before the first evaluation is written and discussed. Ideally, new employees should learn about the evaluation process as soon as they are hired. Their first exposure to the process in action usually takes place at the end of their probationary period, which in most organizations is 90 days.

Performance evaluations should be part of an ongoing process so you have an idea of the employee's progress at all times. Waiting until a full year has elapsed before evaluating employees is a disservice to you and to them. It's best to meet with each employee at least quarterly so you can review areas of weakness and provide encouragement toward agreed-upon goals.

Discipline

Over the last decade, the trend for dealing with employees who perform below expectations is "positive" discipline. In this process, you follow a defined progression from unwritten oral counseling to extensively documented criteria that the employee must agree to if he or she wants to stay employed. The process is "positive" because it allows employees many opportunities to discuss performance-related issues with you before being terminated. The positive aspect for you, the manager, is that if you have followed the process faithfully it protects you and the business from legal liability for wrongful termination.

The key to disciplining employees is to follow the process consistently and to document each event in the employee's file as it happens. Discipline should never be a surprise. Each employee should know the expectations of the job and be alerted if he or she is not measuring up. When you document underachievement, state only objective facts. For example, saying "you are not performing up to par" is subjective, but saying "last month you performed only 5 drug therapy problem interventions and our target is at least 10," is objective.

Discipline employees as soon as they perform below expectations; do not wait for their annual evaluation. Most large organizations separate the discipline process from the performance evaluation process to allow employees an opportunity to improve before their formal evaluation. Let the employee state his or her views on the issue and document them in their permanent file. Together, decide how the employee's performance will improve, when the next evaluation will occur, and what happens if no progress is made.

Operations

Dispensing functions and patient care are intimately linked. How can you improve medication-related outcomes without the patient receiving the correct medication? In policy and procedure manuals, however, the dispensing and patient care functions are separate and distinct parts of the operations section.

The dispensing portion of the manual will be easier to construct than the patient care section because pharmacists are intimately familiar with dispensing tasks and they are easily compartmentalized. In each section, include specific resources and training options to help ensure that employees are able to perform competently.

In the operations section on patient services, spell out such activities as pharmacy and therapeutics (P&T) committee, drug use evaluation, adverse drug reaction reporting, pharmacokinetics, patient education, health screenings, and drug therapy reviews. Specify the hours during which the services are provided and how to contact pharmacists during off hours. Other topics to consider covering are pharmaceutical care, quality assurance and documentation, outcomes measurement, and new program development.

The dispensing section will likely contain both policies and procedures, but the patient services section will probably contain mostly policy statements. Task-oriented patient services such as drug use evaluation and P&T committee support lend themselves to procedures, but face-to-face patient consultation typically does not. Consultations unfold differently each time depending on variables such as the patient's personality, health conditions, and knowledge. For these kinds of activities, it's best to include a policy statement describing what is expected. For example, the statement might say that pharmacists' con-

> **R Common Dispensing-Related Topics in Manuals**
>
> + Ordering and receiving medication inventory.
> + Accounting for and dispensing controlled substances.
> + Procedures for handling, storing, and preparing intravenous drug products.
> + Dispensing prescription medications to outpatients or employees.
> + Processing and delivering inpatient medication orders.
> + Filling carts or servicing automated dispensing machines.
> + Hours of pharmacy service.
> + Procedures for dispensing and distributing medications when the computer is down.
> + Reference or resource list (formulary, etc.)
> + Rules, regulations, statutes, etc.

sultations aim to identify and resolve drug-related problems. Patient services that typically require both a policy statement and a description of procedures are medication history taking, pharmacokinetic monitoring, patient education, and disease-state management.

Continuous Quality Improvement

Today, many organizations are adding sections on continuous quality improvement (CQI) to their policy and procedure manuals. See Chapter 10 for an in-depth discussion of CQI.

CQI-related policies and procedures set the stage for how the pharmacy should foster improvement in all areas, including dispensing, patient services, and human resources. In most organizations, CQI follows the rapid-cycle improvement model espoused by the Institute for Healthcare Improvement (see http://www.IHI.org). With rapid-cycle improvement, you quickly make small but substantive changes in each process until it improves. You then maintain the process at its improved state until it requires another rapid cycle because performance drops below a certain standard. Policies and procedures are very helpful in spelling out how to maintain improvements or enhance them.

Tips for Great Manuals

If you feel daunted by the prospect of compiling or revising your policies and procedures, you're not alone. The tips below should enable you to think through the process and develop a user-friendly manual that helps your staff be productive and your pharmacy operate smoothly. So that your manual is easy to update, use three-ring binders with tabbed section dividers.

1 . Place yourself in the role of a new employee, or have a new employee review your policies and procedures manual. Ask one question: "If you need to understand how to operate this business or department, could you find the information in the manual?"

2 . Never create a policy and procedure manual or add a new section in the heat of the moment. Always ask yourself why the document is being created before you write it. If the problem you're addressing is small, deal with it outside of a written document.

3 . Put a purpose statement on each policy and procedure. This helps clarify the issue at hand and allows users to determine quickly if the section will answer their question or help them solve a problem.

4 . Place the date that the policy or procedure was first enacted, along with the date of last revision, on top of the policy or procedure document.

5 . Plan to review and revise your policies and procedures manual every other year. Schedule reviews and revisions just as you would schedule periodic inventories, accreditation visits, or regulatory evaluations. Discard those parts of the manual that are no longer useful.

6 . Get input from employees to determine the best way to organize the manual.

7 . Keep policies and procedures as short as possible so they are useful and easy to grasp.

8 . Involve your staff in writing new or updating old policies and procedures. If your staff does not have the time, skills, or interest for this task, be sure they review and critique anything new before it is enacted.

9 . Maintain an accurate table of contents so information can always be retrieved easily.

Using Space Effectively

It's a given that pharmacies must be set up to meet legal and regulatory requirements for the security and safety of employees, patients, and the drug inventory. Beyond that, your physical environment should promote patient care and help staff work more efficiently.

Closely examine the ideal practice you described at the beginning of this chapter and the related flow diagrams you developed. Then estimate how much space you need for your practice activities. Many sources, including *A Practical Guide to Pharmaceutical Care*,[10] give guidance on re-engineering your pharmacy layout and workflow. The Department of Defense pharmacy space standards (http://www.va.gov/facmgt/standard/dguide/pharm/pharm06.pdf) and the Department of Veterans' Affairs planning criteria for VA facilities (http://www.va.gov/vha-fp/space) give detailed breakdowns of pharmacy space requirements and reasonable estimates of the space needed for each component of pharmacy practice. They also contain information to help you justify your space needs. Below are angles to consider as you evaluate your physical environment.

+ **Positive work life.** Most people devote a great deal of time and effort to making their home safe and comfortable, yet they spend most of their waking hours at the workplace. Although there are restrictions on how much you can change your work environment, giving it a more pleasant feel contributes to job satisfaction— which in turn translates to efficient and effective performance.
+ **Customer perception.** As the old saying goes, "You never get a second chance to make a first impression." When patients, physicians, nurses, or customers walk into a pharmacy that looks cluttered and unkempt, they're not likely to expect a high level of health care services. Patients who see a traditional prescription dispensing area with only "in" and "out" windows are not likely to imagine they could have private counseling sessions with the pharmacist. But if they walk into a neat, well-lit pharmacy with a "physician office" appearance, they will probably expect or be receptive to patient care services.
+ **Workflow.** A patient-oriented practice requires sufficient space so that workflow is smooth for both product-related functions and patient care. Although the two probably overlap, product-related functions have to do mostly with filling prescriptions and patient-related functions involve assessment and counseling. Consider how labor involving these two areas is divided and set things up so pharmacists can easily contribute to the patient workflow and technicians to the product workflow.
+ **Privacy.** To counsel patients and perform assessments, including limited physical exams, you need privacy, which isn't always easy to come by. Privacy is especially difficult to find in retail practices. Keep in mind that privacy does not necessarily mean a separate, completely enclosed room. A private space simply needs to be

secluded enough for the patient to feel comfortable talking about personal health matters.

+ **Space and location.** Space is always an issue, no matter what type of pharmacy you manage. When deciding where to conduct patient-focused activities, be sure to minimize the distance from dispensing and patient waiting areas. Pharmacists need to be able to reach the spot quickly. Patients don't want to feel conspicuous as they make their way to the counseling area.

An outpatient pharmacy based in a hospital or clinic should be in an area with high traffic flow that is convenient to patients as they are leaving. In acute care practices, satellite pharmacies are often well received in patient care units because this arrangement makes pharmacists more accessible to the other health care staff. However, some facilities avoid satellite pharmacies because they compete for valuable floor space and may require more resources to run than a centralized distribution system.

When justifying your space needs, you'll have to explain the pharmacist's role beyond product distribution and the importance of an infrastructure that's conducive to patient care. Unfortunately, space often becomes an emotional "turf" battle. In the institutional setting, those who occupy space (regardless of what they are doing with it) may be reluctant to give it up for fear of needing it in the future. In community or retail settings, space for creating a patient consultation area often conflicts with space for inventory or merchandise.

Conclusion

Infrastructure is a critical, but often overlooked, component of pharmacy practice. The right infrastructure allows the drug use process to flow smoothly and makes it possible to provide cost-effective, high-quality patient services. To be sure you have the right infrastructure for your needs, you must clearly understand what you want to accomplish and research the options available.

Among key components of infrastructure are automation, space planning, use of technicians, and development of policies and procedures that address all aspects of the pharmacy operation. It's important to have a work environment that merges function with aesthetics so that staff function efficiently and patients feel good about coming into your pharmacy.

References

1. Johnson JA, Bootman JL. Drug related morbidity and mortality: a cost of illness model. *Arch Intern Med*. 1995;155:1949-56.
2. Hepler CD, Strand LM. Opportunities and responsibilities in pharmaceutical care. *Am J Hosp Pharm*. 1990;47:533-43.
3. Holland RW, Nimmo CM. Transitions in pharmacy practice part 3: effecting change–the three-ring circus. *Am J Health Syst Pharm*. 1999:56:2235-41.
4. Covey SR. *The Seven Habits of Highly Effective People*. New York: Simon and Shuster; 1989.
5. O'Malley CH. Pharmacy and the e-train: time to get on board (editorial). *Am J Health Syst Pharm*. 2001;58:39.
6. Nickman NA, Guerrero RM, Bair JN. Self-reported work-sampling methods for evaluating pharmaceutical services. *Am J Hosp Pharm*. 1990;47:1611-17.
7. Schumock GT, Meet PD, Ploetz PA, et al. Economic evaluations of clinical pharmacy services–1988-1995. The publications committee of the American College of Clinical Pharmacy. *Pharmacotherapy*. 1996;16:1188-1208.
8. ASHP Patient Concerns Survey Research Report, September 1999. Available at: http://www.ashp.org/public/public_relations/survey.html. Accessed June 1, 2001.
9. Mutnick AH, Sterba KJ, Peroutka JA, et al. Cost savings and avoidance from clinical interventions. *Am J Health Syst Pharm*. 1997:54:392-6.
10. Rovers JP, Currie JD, Hagel HP, et al. *A Practical Guide to Pharmaceutical Care*. Washington, DC: American Pharmaceutical Association; 1998:119-27.

Chapter 5
MOTIVATING STAFF FOR PATIENT CARE
Christine M. Nimmo & Ross W. Holland

When introducing pharmaceutical care, getting your staff on board is essential. In fact, your success or failure hinges on it. Without staff who can and want to make the change, all the best equipment, computerization, private consultation areas, and marketing plans in the world will mean nothing.

Two critical issues are addressed in this chapter to help you facilitate a change in practice: How do you get existing staff to willingly change from a distributive practice model to pharmaceutical care, and how do you select new staff for this role?

This chapter refers to health-system pharmacists and community pharmacists. The former term includes traditional hospital inpatient pharmacy practice, outpatient clinic pharmacy, long-term care, managed care, home care, and other aspects of pharmacy practice that are part of an organized health care system. The latter term refers to traditional chain or independently owned community pharmacies that are not formally part of any health care system or network.

The Pharmaceutical Care Pharmacist

Having competent pharmacists is critical to providing pharmaceutical care. That's why it is essential to understand what constitutes competence in pharmaceutical care before putting this practice in place. According to the Professional Competence Equation shown in Figure 5-1, three sets of competencies characterize a person professionally competent in a given area of practice: skills, professional socialization, and judgment.[1-4] In fact, the Professional Competence Equation is written as an algebraic equation to signify that the person is professionally competent only when all three components are present.

Skills

The skills component encompasses psychomotor skills, such as the manipulative skills required in compounding, and intellectual problem-solving skills, which require both knowledge of the pertinent content and possession of the thinking strategy

The publisher wishes to acknowledge the American Society of Health-System Pharmacists for the contribution of this chapter, © American Society of Health-System Pharmacists, Inc.

Figure 5-1. Professional Competence Equation

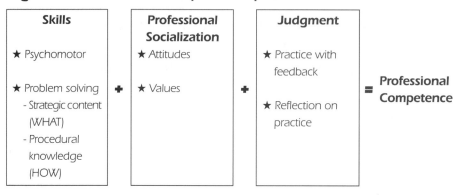

required for solving the problem. Examples of intellectual problem-solving skills include the ability to apply the results of a particular clinical study to the design of a patient's medication regimen, and the communications strategies necessary to elicit pertinent patient information.

Professional Socialization

The second component—professional socialization—reflects the professional values and attitudes associated with the practice model. This aspect of professional competence determines how the practitioner answers questions such as:

* What social values do I serve in my work?
* Who am I ultimately responsible to in my work?
* What are appropriate job responsibilities for me as a pharmacist?
* What should be my relationship to other health care providers?
* What should be the nature of my relationship to patients?
* What is my responsibility to the profession of pharmacy?

The answers to these questions determine the practitioner's day-by-day choice of activities and the priority set on these activities.

Judgment

Judgment is the third feature of the professionally competent person. In pharmacy, this is the ability of seasoned practitioners to routinely make sound decisions in complex problem situations. Practitioners may speak of this ability as "my intuition" or "my gut feeling." Practitioners who achieve the competencies of judgment do so through extensive experience and by constantly reflecting on what they are doing, evaluating how well it does or doesn't work, and learning what will improve their performance.

What Constitutes Competence?

What makes a pharmacist competent within any of the practice models that constitute pharmacy today? The skills required for professional competence vary among models.[3] Table 5-1 contrasts the knowledge and skills required in the distributive and pharmaceutical care practice models. Table 5-2 contrasts the professional values and attitudes of the distributive and pharmaceutical care pharmacist. The judgment component of professional competence also varies among models of practice. Consequently, the judgment of a distributive pharmacist may have little to do with the judgment of a pharmaceutical care pharmacist.

The Practice Change Model

Many managers have tried to transform their departments or pharmacies to the practice of pharmaceutical care, with varying levels of success. The change models and workplace motivational theories they've used have proven to be unsatisfactory guides in pharmacy's unique change situation. The problem is that these resources tend to focus on one thing—increasing the pharmacist's knowledge about a topic. They overlook the fact that an appropriate practice environment and a well-motivated pharmacist are also necessary if change is to be successful. The Holland-Nimmo Practice Change Model (PCM)[3,5-8] helps managers focus on all three areas that must be addressed when transforming a pharmacy practice.*

 The Professional Competence Equation Describes Skills

The Professional Competence Equation describes the skills of a pharmacist professionally competent in pharmaceutical care. These competencies include:

+ Intellectual problem-solving skills.
+ Values and attitudes.
+ Clinical judgment associated with direct patient care.

Christine Nimmo's work on the Practice Change Model (PCM) is conducted through the American Society of Health-System Pharmacists (ASHP), which has authorized the use of the model via educational presentations and workshops.

 Contrasts in Clinical Judgment

The distributive pharmacist seeking professional competence reflects on problems concerning the preparation and distribution of medications. Will this medication remain stable in the patient's home refrigerator? Is the patient allergic to this newly prescribed medication?

The pharmaceutical care pharmacist seeking professional competence reflects on problems concerning the direct care of patients. How do I help this patient with diabetes see the importance of insulin monitoring? What dose of this antiemetic would be the best choice for this patient with cancer undergoing chemotherapy?

Table 5-1. Knowledge and Skills Competencies Associated with the Distributive and Pharmaceutical Care Practice Models

In the Distributive Practice Model, pharmacists:

+ Ensure the completeness of a medication order before preparing or permitting distribution of the first dose.
+ Interpret the appropriateness of a medication order before preparing or permitting distribution of the first dose.
+ Follow established policies and procedures to maintain the accuracy of the patient profile.
+ Prepare medication products by using appropriate techniques and following established policies and procedures.
+ Dispense medication by following established policies and procedures.
+ Provide basic medication use information to patients.
+ Follow accepted policies and procedures to document medication distribution activities.

In the Pharmaceutical Care Practice Model, pharmacists:

+ Use the skills of empathy and assertiveness to establish caring, collaborative relationships with patients and their other health care providers.
+ Use effective drug literature evaluation skills to satisfy patient questions related to the design of therapy.
+ Collect and organize all patient-specific information needed to prevent, detect, and resolve medication-related problems and make appropriate therapeutic recommendations.
+ Determine the presence of existing and potential medication and related therapeutic problems.
+ Develop pharmacotherapeutic and related health care goals with the patient or caregiver that integrate patient-specific data, disease-specific and drug-specific information, and ethical and quality-of-life considerations.
+ Design or modify an existing therapeutic regimen so that it meets the goals established for the patient; integrates patient-specific disease and drug information, ethical issues, and quality-of-life issues; and considers pharmacoeconomic principles.
+ Collaborate with the patient or caregiver to design or modify an existing monitoring plan that effectively evaluates achievement of pharmacotherapeutic and related health care goals.
+ Confirm the care plan for the patient with pertinent members of the patient care team.
+ Use approved procedures to implement a care plan that addresses how medication will be administered and which laboratory tests and monitoring approaches will be needed.
+ Modify the care plan as necessary on the basis of monitoring data.
+ Effectively use evidence-based biomedical literature to defend patient care decisions, when necessary.
+ Demonstrate responsibility for the outcomes of patient care by consistently advocating the patient's health and well-being.
+ Use effective patient education techniques to provide counseling to patients and caregivers, including information on drug therapy, adverse effects, compliance, appropriate use, handling, and medication administration.

Table 5-2. Professional Values and Attitudes Associated with Distributive and Pharmaceutical Care Practice Models

Question Answered by Professional Values and Attitudes	Response Associated with the Distributive Model	Response Associated with the Pharmaceutical Care Model
What social values do I serve in my work?	Ensure that the right drug is received by the right patient at the right time	Ensure that the desired health care outcomes for the patient are achieved
To whom am I as a pharmacist ultimately responsible in my work?	The prescriber	The patient
What are appropriate job responsibilities for me as a pharmacist?	Prepare and distribute drug products; provide information on use	Design, recommend, monitor, and evaluate patient-specific pharmacotherapy
What should be my relationship with other health care providers?	Support the prescriber's goals; limited or nonexistent relationship with other health care providers	Collaborate in the decision-making process regarding the patient's medication therapy
What should be the nature of my relationship with patients?	Limited; provide a product and focused technical information	Collaborative, caring relationship; assist with patient problem-solving
What is my responsibility to the profession of pharmacy?	1. Accept responsibility and accountability for membership in the profession 2. Engage in lifelong learning relevant to one's area of practice 3. Actively commit to the *Oath of a Pharmacist* and *Code of Ethics for Pharmacists* 4. Dedicate to practice excellence 5. Maintain highest ideals and professional attributes	1. Accept responsibility and accountability for membership in the profession 2. Engage in lifelong learning relevant to one's area of practice 3. Actively commit to the *Oath of a Pharmacist* and *Code of Ethics for Pharmacists* 4. Dedicate to practice excellence 5. Maintain highest ideals and professional attributes

The PCM is a leadership tool for maximizing the possibility that a pharmacist will actually make a significant change in practice and move to pharmaceutical care. As shown in Figure 5-2, it has three leadership components that the manager must simultaneously satisfy to optimize the probability of change. These components, which are explained in the next few pages, are:

+ Practice environment.
+ Learning resources.
+ Motivational strategies.

Figure 5-2. The Holland-Nimmo Practice Change Model (PCM)

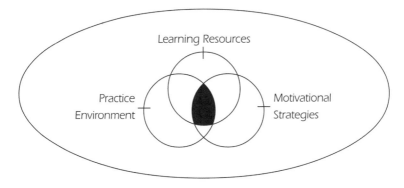

First, Develop Operational Statements

We cannot overemphasize the importance of completing this step before applying the Practice Change Model. Developing operational statements prompts everyone involved to think about exactly the same change and the specific tasks involved. Clarity of purpose is essential—to the manager, those in power and authority, and those called upon to change. Base your operational statements on the mission and vision statements you created in Chapters 1 and 2. The operational statements should be developed by your guiding coalition (see page 32) and may take up several pages, in contrast to your vision statement, which is usually only a paragraph or two.

Each operational statement should describe, in very concrete terms, what you want each staff member to start doing. Word this statement so that it communicates the change exactly to all audiences involved. Vague statements such as, "I want all staff to provide pharmaceutical care to our patients," will not suffice because they don't convey the exact changes required of each employee. Instead, be specific. Develop an individualized statement for each staff member who will be required to change. For example: "I want Jeremy, who currently checks all orders received for completeness, prepares the medications for distribution, and counsels patients on their medication use (which falls within the distribution model), to collaborate with the patient and other members of the health care team in designing, recommending, monitoring, and evaluating pharmacotherapy for patients with hyperlipidemia (which falls within the pharmaceutical care model)."

This statement names the person to change and describes the practitioner's current practice responsibilities and the practice model into which they fall. It also describes the tasks to be assumed and the practice model into which *they* fall. This laser-clear goal will subsequently govern activities in all three components of the model. You will use it to coordinate changes necessary in the practice environment, to acquire learning resources, and to create motivational strategies.

For the purposes of this chapter we will simply refer to the envisioned new role as the "desired practice."

Your goal may be as narrow as providing pharmaceutical care to manage just one disease state or as broad as addressing all disease states. The service you want to provide may be limited to just one age group or may apply to your entire patient population. No matter the scope, your goal must be precise and worded so that all the staff involved can understand it.

Step One: Create a Conducive Practice Environment

The first leadership component of the Practice Change Model is creating an environment in which the pharmacist can actually perform the envisioned tasks. Creating an environment receptive to change involves removing or minimizing all significant barriers to full implementation of the desired practice. As Figure 5-3 shows, this hierarchical process begins with societal, moves to health system (in health-system practice) or corporate/owner (in community practice), and concludes with practice site-level stumbling blocks.

Figure 5-3. Practice Environment

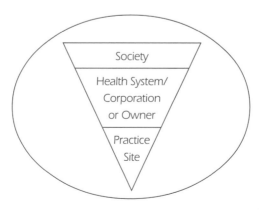

Societal Barriers

Whether you are a health-system or community practice manager with change in mind, you will face these potential societal barriers:*

+ Do federal, state, and local laws and regulations permit the desired practice?
+ Do the potential patients accept the service provided by pharmacists in the desired practice?
+ At the national level, do the other health care professions accept the desired practice as part of the role of the pharmacist?

As a manager, your first task in creating a conducive practice environment is to use these three questions to identify any societal level barriers that will hinder the establishment of an accepting environment. Next, you should generate a strategy for minimizing or removing each significant barrier. You must also resolve significant societal level barriers or there is no point in proceeding to the second level of barrier identification and resolution.

Health-System or Community Practice Barriers

At this next level of barrier identification and resolution, you will find variations depending on whether you are in health-system or community practice. Further, you will encounter variations within community practice depending on whether your pharmacy is totally independent or part of a larger corporation. The following diagnostic questions—which include all possible environments—can help you identify potential health-system and community pharmacy barriers.

+ Are there any health-system administrators or corporate executives whose support you will need for the desired practice and who are not currently convinced of the desired change?
+ Are there any health-system or corporate reporting relationships that may hinder adoption of the desired practice?
+ Are there any inadequacies in the pharmacy's physical facilities that would hinder establishment of the desired practice?
+ Are there any financial resources that you will require to establish the desired practice?
+ Are there any additions to staff or changes in staffing patterns that you will require to establish the desired practice?
+ Are there any other health care professionals in the health system or community whose support you will need but who do not currently understand the need for the desired practice?

The authors of this chapter wish to acknowledge the contributions of the following ASHP members to the development of the list of potential practice environment barriers: Richard L. Lucarotti, PharmD; Juan J. Martinez, MS; Kay Ryan, MS; and Michael D. Sanborn, MS.

✦ Are there any limitations in the health system's or corporation's use of technology (e.g., information systems, robotics) that would hinder establishment of the desired practice?
✦ Is union support required for approval of the desired practice?
✦ Are there any human resources management restrictions that would hinder establishment of the desired practice?
✦ Are there any limitations to accessing information pertinent to the desired practice (e.g., physician-based medical records, medication errors, patient profiles, adverse drug reactions, length of stay)?
✦ Are there any health-system or corporate policy constraints on pharmacist practice activities that may hinder the establishment of the desired practice (e.g.,writing in the chart, ordering laboratory tests)?

Just like with societal level barriers, you must identify which barriers exist and determine if their strength can derail the establishment of a practice environment conducive to the desired practice. For each significant barrier, you must implement a strategy to minimize or remove it before you can successfully move to identifying significant barriers and strategies at the practice site level.

Practice Site Barriers

Unlike societal and health-system barriers, practice site barriers are directly under your control and are probably more amenable to correction. Use the following questions to determine potential barriers at the practice site level:

✦ Are there any patterns in the pharmacy's workflow that would hinder establishment of the desired practice?
✦ Are there discrepancies surrounding the existing professional relationship between the pharmacist and each affected member of the health care team and the relationship required for successful establishment of the desired practice?
✦ Are there any financial, staffing, and time implications that will affect staff training requirements for the desired practice?
✦ Are there differences between the pharmacist's current job description and a job description that accurately describes the pharmacist's desired practice?
✦ Are there differences in the present pharmacy staff's norms, values, and expectations about practice and those that are required to support the desired practice?

When you have identified and minimized or removed all significant barriers to establishing the desired practice, your leadership tasks are complete. At this point you can begin the managerial tasks of actually implementing the desired practice. These managerial tasks are described in later chapters of this book.

Step Two: Provide the Required Learning Resources

As the preceding discussion of professional competence illustrates, competence in pharmaceutical care involves its own set of intellectual problem-solving skills and clinical judgment. Most likely, a pharmacist who has routinely engaged in distribution will not possess the skills, competencies, or clinical judgment that comprise pharmaceutical care competence. The second leadership component of the Practice Change Model requires the manager to ensure that learning needs are identified and met. Figure 5-4 illustrates the requirements for meeting the learning resources component.

Figure 5-4. Learning Resources

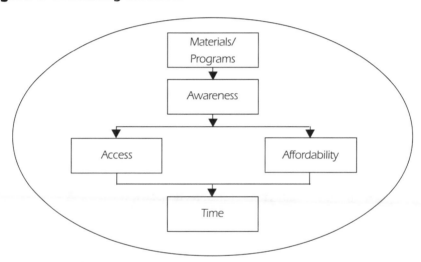

Identify Appropriate Learning Resources

Initially, you must ensure that the appropriate learning resources exist to meet the pharmacist's needs. You will need to systematically diagnose learning needs and accurately assess what kinds of training will produce the desired learning outcomes. To accomplish this task, you must satisfactorily answer the following questions:

- Have the knowledge, skills, and abilities required to perform each of the desired practice activities been identified?
- Has each practitioner been assessed to determine missing knowledge, skills, and abilities required for performance of the desired practice activities?
- Are the practitioners informed of the learning assessment results?
- Have the identified learning needs been converted into educational objectives according to a learning taxonomy[9-11] to determine whether existing materials and

programs will produce the required learning outcomes? (A learning taxonomy describes the sequence of steps by which someone learns a new fact, skill, or attitude.)

+ Do instructional resources include the selection of teaching methods that will achieve the desired level of learning?

Ensure Access, Affordability, and Commitment

As a manager, you cannot stop at simply identifying satisfactory learning resources. If the practitioner is charged with securing all or part of the learning resources, he or she must be knowledgeable of alternative sources that will fulfill the need. You must also consider issues of practicality. First, of the existing learning resources that will fulfill the learning need, which are geographically accessible and offered at a time when the practitioner can use them? Second, are they affordable? Additional points to consider include:

+ What is the total cost to complete the required learning?
+ Are any funds allocated by the health system, corporation, or owner for the change in practice currently available?
+ Is there a well-designed plan for the use of health-system, corporate, or owner funds for training for the desired practice?
+ Will the practitioner be required to fund all or part of his or her training?
+ Has the practitioner committed to his or her portion of the training costs?
+ Is there time for the practitioner to do the necessary study?
+ If the employer is committed to providing time for the required learning, have issues related to making that time available been resolved?
+ If the pharmacist is committed to providing time for the required learning, has he or she resolved issues related to making that time available?

As the leader of the change process, the manager must achieve satisfactory answers to all the questions raised in the learning resources component. Appropriateness, affordability, access, and time are all critical pieces. Locating existing programs that can meet these criteria will surely involve researching educational resources from a number of providers in a variety of formats (e.g., lectures, workshops, written materials, CD-ROMs) and delivery mechanisms (e.g., live presentations, Web-based training, teleconferencing). In many cases, you may have to customize an existing program for it to meet the specific training needs of the staff or an individual.

After performing the requirements of this component, the pharmacy leader will have an effective and efficient training plan to meet the individual training needs of each pharmacist involved in change. Chapter 6, as well as the ASHP publication *Staff Development for Pharmacy Practice*,[4] further address training issues.

Step Three: Motivate the Person to Change

The model's third leadership responsibility is to motivate the person to do any required learning and then engage in the desired practice. As a first step, the manager must decide if the pharmacist is driven by professional values or if this person simply regards his or her practice as a "job." The motivational approach offered in this chapter applies strictly to the "professional" pharmacist. You can find the appropriate approach for those with the "it's just a job" orientation in traditional managerial literature on workplace motivation. But remember, no matter which orientation characterizes the practitioner you want to change, you must fully address and satisfy the motivational component.

For the professional pharmacist, your leadership task is to employ motivational strategies that generate an intense desire in the person to practice pharmaceutical care, the belief that he or she is capable of doing so, and commitment to a plan to attain any necessary knowledge, skill, or clinical judgment to engage in the desired practice.

The Practice Change Model advocates that the most promising route to motivating change in a professional person is through professional resocialization. This approach is based on Festinger's Theory of Cognitive Dissonance,[12] which asserts that when someone's belief system is out of sync with his or her actions, it produces such emotional discomfort that the person will change behavior in order to restore internal harmony.

Traditional workplace motivational tools, such as money and promotion, should not be entirely overlooked. However, in today's cost-cutting health care atmosphere, money and promotion are scarce or nonexistent commodities. More importantly, most pharmacists are professionals—people driven to do what they do each day by a set of values and attitudes about the purpose and responsibilities of their practices. For a professional person, real change—the kind that sticks when the manager isn't looking and places the pharmacist firmly in the pharmaceutical care practice model—is rooted in the adoption of the attitudes and values of pharmaceutical care.

Before you introduce the training identified in the learning resources component, you must first instill in the pharmacist the desire to engage in pharmaceutical care. Then, you must make the

Motivating Pharmacists to Change Their Practice

For the professional pharmacist, your leadership task is to employ motivational strategies that generate:

+ An intense desire in the individual to practice pharmaceutical care.
+ The belief that he or she is capable of doing so.
+ Commitment to a plan to attain any necessary knowledge, skill, or clinical judgment to engage in the desired practice.

pharmacist believe that it is something he or she can do, and get him or her to commit to a plan for attaining required learning. This strategy will produce the intrinsic motivation for practice change and a learner with a higher degree of motivation to practice pharmaceutical care. Until this is achieved, the effects of a training program are likely to be greatly diminished. Put simply, the unmotivated learner is a poor learner. Figure 5-5 illustrates the relationship between mindset, motivation, and change. Change only occurs in motivated pharmacists—and to become motivated, they must start with the right mindset.

Figure 5-5. Motivation and Change

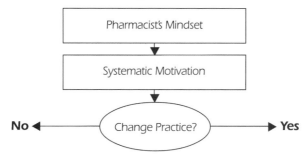

The manager who employs this strategy of intrinsic motivation for change is actually engaged in the process of teaching. The Nimmo-Holland Motivational Guide for Practice Change (see Table 5-3, page 108) adapts Krathwohl's Taxonomy for the Affective Domain[10]—the educational community's guidebook for teaching values and attitudes—to the unique changes in the practice of pharmacy.

As the Nimmo-Holland Guide shows, the manager must move the practitioner through four learning stages to professionally resocialize him or her to commit to the values and attitudes of pharmaceutical care. In Stage 1, *finding out about it*, the practitioner acquires a solid comprehension of what pharmaceutical care practice is about. In Stage 2, *testing the water*, the practitioner advances to understanding the emotional response he or she will experience by engaging in pharmaceutical care and also begins to see what adoption of the desired practice will involve. In Stage 3, *gaining commitment*, the pharmacist completes the formation of the values and attitudes of pharmaceutical care and gains a strong belief that this is what he or she should do. During Stage 4, *making sure it sticks*, the practitioner reshuffles his or her existing value system to make room for all that is involved in becoming a pharmaceutical care practitioner.

The next section describes how you as the teacher must move the practitioner through the four stages of acquiring the values and attitudes of pharmaceutical care—including what to do, how to do it, and when to do it.

Table 5-3. Nimmo-Holland Motivational Guide for Practice Change

Stage	Motivational Activities	Stage Indicators
1. Finding Out About It	✦ Conduct interactive lectures/guided discussions ✦ Encourage informal discussions with colleagues ✦ Call attention to articles ✦ Invite near-peer role models on-site ✦ Conduct site visits to near-peers ✦ Discuss WIIFM (What's in it for me?) ✦ Brainstorm barriers to adoption	1.1 "I'm aware that some pharmacists do those things, but couldn't care less about it." 1.2 "Well, I guess it's possible for pharmacists to do that." 1.3 "This idea about practice intrigues me." 1.4 "I've been told I must learn more about this new kind of practice. I do what I'm told."
2. Testing the Water	✦ Provide access to near-peers in this type of practice ✦ Try out on a partial basis ✦ Make them feel competent ✦ Provide feedback	2.1 "I'm interested in learning more about this new kind of practice." 2.2 "I'm enjoying the idea of playing around with this new kind of practice."
3. Gaining Commitment	✦ Continue access to near-peers in this type of practice ✦ Create opportunities to publicly identify with this practice	3.1 "This type of practice has a place in the role of the pharmacist." 3.2 "If you gave me a choice, I believe I'd choose this type of practice." 3.3 "I am firmly convinced this kind of practice is what I should be doing."
4. Making Sure It Sticks	✦ Encourage verbalization of practice concept to others ✦ Provide access to near-peers who have retrained for this practice	4.1 "Let me tell you how when a pharmacist practices this way, all the bases for a pharmacist's contribution to patient care are covered." 4.2 "I have a plan for learning the new skills I need to do this kind of practice, and I'm committed to using some of my personal time to do it."

Stage 1: Finding Out About It

The logic of Stage 1 learning is simple. A practitioner can't think clearly or make an intelligent decision about whether to pursue the manager's desired practice without having an accurate, concrete understanding of what that practice is and what he or she would actually be doing. Just think of how the term "pharmaceutical care" has been redefined, reinterpreted, used, and abused since Hepler and Strand[14] introduced it in 1990. Even well-read people and association "groupies" get confused about what it means. Now imagine the potential for misunderstanding by the pharmacist who doesn't read the literature, does not belong to even the local pharmacy association, hasn't been out visiting other pharmacies or health-system pharmacy departments with progressive practices, and who probably only talks pharmacy with people he or she works with—other practitioners who are probably in the same boat. "Finding out about it" is a very real learning task that the manager must address.

How can the manager accomplish this? One way is to convene a discussion group of all the staff members who are slated for change, where you can create an in-depth understanding of the desired practice. It will be critical for pharmacists to focus on learning about the desired practice, so remove them from the immediate work environment, intercoms, and pagers.

Ideally, the leader should be a near-peer. Begin with an interactive lecture that includes the presentation of ideas interspersed with focused questions to help the group clarify their understanding. Follow this with a guided discussion of carefully structured questioning to further help participants arrive at a correct

 The Four Learning Stages of Change

+ Stage 1: Finding out about it.
+ Stage 2: Testing the water.
+ Stage 3: Gaining commitment.
+ Stage 4: Making sure it sticks.

 The Influence of a Near-Peer

Well-respected literature on the diffusion of innovations,[13] which describes how change is gradually adopted, reveals that there is a powerful positive influence on adopting change when people perceive that the advocate is someone similar to them. Thus, a village woman is most likely to adopt birth control practices when another woman in the same village encourages her, and a physician is most likely to change treatment of a disease when a respected fellow practitioner says she's tried the new way and achieved good outcomes. By extrapolation, the most effective change advocate of pharmaceutical care practice for a BS pharmacist who has long labored at distribution is another BS pharmacist who once practiced distribution and now successfully engages in pharmaceutical care. For this reason, it is helpful to use near-peers, whenever possible, in your teaching activities.

conceptual picture of the desired practice. Principles to follow for the discussion group include the following:

- The discussion leader's presentation should attempt to connect the practitioner's current practice model with pharmaceutical care by stressing similarities as well as differences. In this way, the practitioner will not perceive pharmaceutical care as completely disassociated from his or her current attitudes and values about practice.
- Present pharmaceutical care in a simplified version that is totally clear to the practitioner.
- Present the idea with concrete application to real situations that the pharmacist encounters and understands.
- Add concreteness to the description of pharmaceutical care by having the pharmacists construct a hypothetical day at work for a practitioner engaged in the model.
- People who absorb "how to" knowledge but not a knowledge of the principles underlying a practice change are in greater danger of misusing the new idea and ultimately discontinuing it than persons who see the full picture. Consequently, it is important at this early stage to address the philosophical issues of practice that underlie pharmaceutical care.
- The discussion leader must sufficiently clarify the contrast between what the practitioner is currently doing and what is desired. This will eliminate any possibility that the practitioner will leave the discussion thinking, "I've always done this."
- In the group discussion the leader must ensure that everyone present engages in the dialogue. Otherwise, there is no assurance that participants have paid attention or have achieved a basic understanding.

After the discussion, the manager can follow up with on-the-job opportunities for practitioners to learn more about the desired practice. For example, the manager can:

- Encourage informal discussion among colleagues centered on the model.
- Call attention to articles that discuss pharmaceutical care.
- Provide opportunities for the practitioner to observe others who engage in this type of practice. If this is not possible in-house, arrange for a field trip or two to another pharmacy where it is being practiced.
- Discuss "What's in it for me?" with the practitioner.
- Where possible, offer external rewards for change such as increased pay, increased job status, choice of work schedule, peer approval, and recognition. These rewards will certainly factor into a person's consideration of "What do I have to gain by doing this?" The manager will also want to call attention to applicable internal rewards such as professional satisfaction, sense of achievement, recognition, and job security.

If the manager successfully brings the practitioner through Stage 1 learning, the practitioner will accurately conceptualize the desired practice, but have no formed judgment about whether or not it is a good thing. The motivational guide in Table 5-3 lists a sequence of observations a practitioner may offer as he or she moves from simple awareness that this type of practice exists to understanding what it is. This list may help the manager judge his or her level of success in achieving Stage 1 learning.

Stage 2: Testing the Water

"Does it fit me? Would it feel good if I did it?" In Stage 2, testing the water, the practitioner learns answers to these questions. The learning going on at this stage is at a personal level. Stage 1 took care of the facts. Now the facts are applied to the self. The would-be downhill skier has read the books, and is now thinking about how she will have to manage that heavy equipment, her love of the outside, her fear of heights, and her passion for speed. The would-be pharmaceutical care practitioner is pondering his present contentment with being in complete control of his work responsibilities, his desire for some intellectual challenge, his dislike of getting involved in other people's emotions, and a desire to contribute more than just the accurate preparation and distribution of widgets.

As the teacher of Stage 2 learning, the manager must help the practitioner relate the desired practice to the practitioner's current value system, interests, and capabilities. It is a time of personal exploration that requires getting as close to the realities of the desired practice as possible. Ideally, the practitioner should shadow a near-peer practitioner of pharmaceutical care for a day or two to get a close look at what the practice is like. The testing can even go as far as attempting one or two of the tasks—in a no-risk situation—to increase the sense of what it would feel like. If the manager cannot arrange an in-house shadowing experience or a field trip for shadowing at another pharmacy, an acceptable alternative is to bring in a near-peer pharmaceutical care practitioner to engage in a discussion of, "This is what my workday is like, and this is what I feel like when I practice this way." Here the practitioner gets a chance to experience pharmaceutical care vicariously.

Your teaching is not complete until the practitioner has experienced positive or negative emotions about engaging in the desired practice. At the end of this stage, if the emotions generated are positive, the impetus to learn more about adopting the desired practice switches from external (at the behest of the manager) to internal (the practitioner's own drive to learn about and consider this practice himself/herself). As illustrated in the motivational guide in Table 5-3, the pharmacist's typical responses will progress from compliance to pleasure.

Stage 3: Gaining Commitment

As the pharmacist moves into Stage 3 of acquiring the attitudes and values of pharmaceutical care, an internal argument ensues. "Is this what I want to do, or isn't it?" The "yes, but" syndrome appears. This is not an argument with the manager or an argument with coworkers. It is a settling with self of private hesitations and uncertainties. The desired outcome of Stage 3 learning is a resolute, "I want to change to a pharmaceutical care practice, and I believe I am capable of doing it."

If Stage 3 learning is an internal discussion, what can an effective teacher do? Simply give the practitioner a rich environment in which to deliberate, including continued access to near-peers who engage in pharmaceutical care. This gives the practitioner a continuing reality check. One of the ways people toy with commitments is to speak them out loud to others, at first quietly in case it doesn't feel right and retreat is required, but louder and louder as conviction grows. It is as if the speaking feeds the conviction and the conviction feeds the speaking. For people whose thought process works that way, the manager can create opportunities to publicly state the growing conviction that pharmaceutical care is the right choice. Such opportunities can take place at discussions within the department.

Stage 4: Making Sure It Sticks

Stage 4 learning moves the pharmacist from the firm conviction, "This is what I want to do," to the development of a committed plan to achieve that goal. He or she enters this last stage of attitude and value formation with an unresolved conflict. The pharmacist has an existing value system that includes the old model of practice, yet he or she is simultaneously being pulled towards the new model. Until now, priorities in the pharmacist's life have been formulated around personal concerns and professional obligations that accommodate the old kind of practice. If pursuit of the desired practice is to move beyond, "I should do this," the practitioner must adjust his or her value system to accommodate doing whatever is required to attain the goal.

As in the previous stage, revising the value system to commit to the practice of pharmaceutical care involves internal deliberation. The manager as teacher can move this process along by helping the practitioner figure out what must be done and how it can be achieved.

At this point, the manager can move to some of the tasks in the learning resources component of the PCM to introduce the competencies required and help the practitioner assess which skills and judgment competencies they lack. This gives the practitioner an accurate fix on the extent of necessary retraining. It also makes clear to what extent other values such as relationships, physical exercise, and hobbies may have to be reshuffled. Near-peers who have retooled for pharmaceutical care can help devise strategies for fitting things in and act as a role model.

Teaching the Values of Pharmaceutical Care: A Hierarchy

Learning values and attitudes is a hierarchical process. The practitioner cannot leapfrog over Stage 1 or any of the other stages in the process and emerge with new values and attitudes. It's akin to mathematics where the child must learn how to add, subtract, multiply, and divide before tackling algebraic equations.

Will all practitioners require significant time to develop understanding of the desired practice? It depends on what the practitioner already knows. Some will simply need clarification of the particular tasks the manager has in mind. Others may have to start from square one and dispel the notion that distribution is not pharmaceutical care. A good teacher will be sure all ducks are in order before moving from one stage of learning to the next.

The pharmacist who successfully learns the new values of pharmaceutical care emerges at the end of Stage 4 with the conviction, "I want to do it. I believe I can do it. I've got a plan to get me there!" This person is inner-driven to pursue the goal. Optimistically, the end result of the professional resocialization process is a pharmacist who cannot wait to get started learning, will remain intently focused on learning even when the going is tough, and will be eager to perform the desired practice as quickly as possible. Hallelujah!

The Influence of Personality

The literature suggests that not every pharmacist is a potential provider of pharmaceutical care.[7] That's why a manager who wants to professionally resocialize a practitioner to pharmaceutical care values and attitudes should first consider the mindset of the pharmacist he or she wishes to influence. The person's entering mindset is constructed of two powerful influences—personality and previous professional socialization. As previously discussed, a person can be professionally resocialized. It happens all the time. But changing a person's personality is another story. Personality is relatively stable, and the manager is unlikely to change it. This is important because research shows that people select their life's work based on a perceived match between their own personalities and the personality characteristics drawn upon by the job. The drive is so strong that a match is achieved by 74.6% of men and 72.3% of women ages 21 to 25 and increases to 91% of men and 90% of women ages 61 to 65.[15] In fact, J.L. Holland[16] states that when there is a mismatch between personality and work environment, one can expect "gross dissatisfaction, ineffective coping behavior, and probably leaving the environment."

Research on the personality characteristics of pharmacists shows a personality type dominated by a strong sense of responsibility, conscientiousness, practicality, logic, and in about one practitioner in five, fear of interpersonal communication. This is to be expected. Remember, at the time most current pharmacists self-selected their profession it was viewed as an occupation consisting largely of technical problem solving and limited contact with patients and other health care professionals. When we speculate on the personality characteristics used by a pharmaceutical care practice model, we see the potential for a strong mismatch. Successful pharmaceutical care practitioners draw heavily on many of the personality characteristics not strongly present in the dominant profile of current practitioners such as independent decision-making, original thinking, patience and understanding, and sociability. These are personality characteristics necessary to establishing caring relationships with patients, engaging in complex clinical problem solving, and participating in team decision-making.

Consequently, the manager who seeks to change values and attitudes should be mindful of the person's mindset—both personality and previous professional socialization—and consider a strong personality mismatch with the pharmaceutical care practice model as a potentially insurmountable barrier to change. Those who refuse to change because of their personality must not be regarded as "bad" pharmacists, but rather as choosing not to make themselves miserable or take on a role that they will not be good at. The manager's responsibility, after trying wholeheartedly to change this person's values and attitudes, should be to assist in the pharmacist's exploration of other vocational interests that will be a better match. Realistically, there may not be a role for everyone in a transformed practice environment.

Some managers have sufficient staff and flexibility to create a limited number of positions requiring distribution only. However, many mismatched practitioners tend to quit when faced with the sure reality that they must engage in the desired model of practice. This removes the unpleasant task of firing, but introduces a new problem— where to find a suitable replacement in today's pharmacist-short job market.

Synergy and Timing

As suggested in Figure 5-2, which illustrates the Practice Change Model, the manager who wants to optimize the possibility that staff members will actually make the change to pharmaceutical care must concurrently satisfy all three leadership components. Clearly, a failure in getting a person to change will likely result when the manager introduces an effective training program and motivates the pharmacist to perform pharmaceutical care, but doesn't set up the environment so that he or she can actually do it. Failure is also likely when the practice environment is squared away and an effective training program is put in place, but the manager fails to adequately motivate the practitioner to practice pharmaceutical care. Likewise, the person can be highly motivated and the practice environment ready for the practice of pharmaceutical care, but if he or she cannot access appropriate training, pharmaceutical care practice is unlikely. Managers working with the model must understand that maximizing success hinges on fully satisfying all three components.

It would simplify matters if the manager could focus intently on meeting the requirements of each component one at a time and in a prescribed order. Then, at the magic moment when all steps were complete, the synergy of the model would set in and wonderful things would happen. Unfortunately, many of the activities in the three components are heavily interrelated.

As a result, nightmare situations can arise when managers pay exclusive attention to one component while excluding the others. For instance, what would it be like to have the practice environment completely in shape so that the pharmacist is handed a new position description and the mandate to fill it, but motivation has been set aside until next week and training to the week after that?

Although managers must accept that working through the model is a process that they will create as they go along, here are some general guiding principles:

+ Don't undertake the PCM leadership tasks until the statement of change is written in language that is understandable by all involved parties.
+ Remember that a job description detailing the desired practice tasks is critical to both the learning resources and motivational strategy components. As a result, you may want to jump down to the practice site level of the practice environment component early on and write the job description in order to get other things moving.
+ Scan learning resources that might meet learning needs early on. However, do not make a decision about the content and structure of a person's training program until the competencies required for the job are specified in a written job description, the learning analysis is done, and the person's competencies have been assessed against the job requirements and a list of learning objectives has been developed.
+ Remember that the motivational strategies are aimed at creating a person who wants to adopt pharmaceutical care practice, believes he or she can do it, and has committed to learning how. Therefore, don't start training until the motivational sequence has been successfully completed.
+ Many things can and will be going on at one time.

What About Technicians?

An obvious question arises. Technicians play a key role in transforming a pharmacy to the delivery of pharmaceutical care. More often than not, technicians as well as pharmacists must make significant changes in their practices if the change is to succeed. Can the PCM be applied to practice change for technicians? The answer is yes, as long as the manager applies the three component principles of the PCM. If significant change is required of the technician, the manager must provide a work environment in which the tasks can be performed. If the technician must learn more in order to do the new tasks this must be addressed, and the technicians must also be motivated to learn and to actually do the new work.

When determining how to approach motivation, the manager must ask the same questions about technicians that they asked about pharmacists. Some technicians are highly professional. For them, changing values and attitudes is the right method. For those who view their work as nothing more than "a job," the manager should consult the techniques of traditional workplace motivation.

Principles of Hiring for Pharmaceutical Care Practice

To transform the department or pharmacy's practice to pharmaceutical care, you must hire pharmacists to provide the services. Hiring the right person requires identifying the candidate who is willing and able to deliver pharmaceutical care and who is professionally competent in this practice model. As discussed in the section about the Professional Competence Equation, screening for suitable employees requires a look at skills, values, attitudes, and the presence or absence of clinical judgment associated with pharmaceutical care. But there are also some additional specifics that will enhance standard hiring practices and help maximize your success in hiring the right person for a pharmaceutical care position.

The Job Description

The logical first step in any hiring strategy is to produce a job description that includes the duties and parameters of the job, the level of responsibility and authority intended, and the attributes specific to and considered essential for the required duties. If the pharmacist will be expected to design and implement the pharmaceutical care service as well as perform direct patient care functions, these management tasks must be accounted for in the job description.

The job description must include all the knowledge, skills, attitudes, and abilities required in the practice. A resource for wording the attitudes and values required of a pharmacist who would engage in pharmaceutical care is included in Table 5-2 of this chapter. However, there is no existing checklist for clinical judgment associated with pharmaceutical care, nor is there likely to be one. Instead, the manager must be intimately familiar with the site's practice—including the types of patients, the disease states commonly treated, and the complexity of cases—in order to formulate some notion of the judgment areas required.

Working from a specific and accurate job description will help you to design advertising for the position, lessen the number of applications you receive without the necessary qualifications, provide the foundation for the interview process, and later on serve as the basis for ongoing performance appraisals.

Recruitment Strategy

Start your recruitment strategy by defining your target audience and then considering all potential recruitment resources including placement services, conferences, job markets, networking, and advertisements in journals, newsletters, and newspapers.

Ask your current pharmacists if they have friends, classmates, or colleagues who may be anxious to embrace your new practice model, and contact them. If you have not already done so, develop a relationship with your local college of pharmacy and become a clerkship site for final-year students. When students with particularly strong skills and aptitude come to your pharmacy on rotation, try to recruit them to join your staff after graduation. And don't forget that students who work for you part time as technicians are a prime source of talent, as well.

The Hiring Process

All three components of professional competence are equally important in hiring the right person. A deficiency in any area produces incompetence. Therefore, the hiring process must attend to all three.

Analysis of skills competencies is essential and is addressed in standard management texts. Assessing the presence and extent of clinical judgment is probably best performed by a clinician who possesses clinical judgment in the desired area. Presenting a series of cases to the interviewee and asking him or her to think out loud through the resolution of the case is an effective method for identifying the presence of clinical judgment. The cases selected should pertain to cases the interviewee would encounter as an employee and include details that mandate the use of clinical judgment.

Since a focus on professional socialization may be new to many managers, here is a direct strategy for ascertaining the candidate's values and beliefs about practice. Simply ask the candidate to write a response to each of the six questions listed in Table 5-2. The candidate's answers will constitute his or her professional socialization. If the responses approximate those suggested in Table 5-2 as corresponding with the pharmaceutical care model, the manager may have a good match.

Above all, the lesson of the Professional Competence Equation is that attitudes and values are just as important as skills or clinical judgment. Without the professional socialization to believe in pharmaceutical care, the person is not professionally competent and is therefore undesirable as an employee in the role of pharmaceutical care delivery—no matter what the level of skills or clinical judgment. If you have to make a choice between an applicant with good clinical skills but the wrong attitude and one with the right attitude and poor clinical skills, it is probably better to hire the latter, providing he or she is willing to learn those skills.

Retaining Pharmaceutical Care Practitioners

Untold amounts of skilled effort, patience, time, and resources are invested in and by individual pharmacists in a successful changeover to pharmaceutical care practice. To protect this investment, it's important to retain pharmacists who are doing a good job in their new practice roles.

In addition to the traditional managerial approaches, the manager's goal in any strategy aimed at retaining pharmaceutical care practitioners will be to build commitment to the health system or to the pharmacy. This is because an employee committed to the organization is likely to stay. When attempting to build commitment to the organization, it is particularly important to keep the four aspects of the work environment in mind.[17]

The first aspect of the work environment is the quality of the relationship between the pharmacist and manager. The second is assuring that rewards—things like preference in scheduling, training, recognition, and raises—are equitably and fairly distributed. Third, for younger, single pharmacists a feeling of belonging can have a significant positive effect on organizational commitment. The fourth aspect to consider is that people who are highly involved in their jobs may get so much positive feedback from the work itself that they seem to be less affected than others by the quality of the relationship with their supervisor. This last aspect of the work environment may be particularly effective in building commitment when a practitioner has been professionally resocialized and is given the opportunity to provide pharmaceutical care.

References

1. Holland RW, Nimmo CM. Leadership and team building. *Internat Pharm J.* 1998;12(Sep-Oct):151-5.

2. Holland RW, Nimmo CM. What is professional competence? *Aust Pharm.* 1998; 17(10):702-5.

3. Nimmo CM, Holland RW. Transitions in pharmacy practice, part 2: who does what and why. *Am J Health Syst Pharm.* 1999;56:1981-7.

4. Nimmo CM, Guerrero RM, Greene SA, et al., eds. *Staff Development for Pharmacy Practice.* Bethesda, MD: American Society of Health-System Pharmacists; 2000.

5. Holland RW, Nimmo CM. Transitions in pharmacy practice, part 1: beyond pharmaceutical care. *Am J Health Syst Pharm.* 1999;56:1758-64.

6. Holland RW, Nimmo CM. Transitions in pharmacy practice, part 3: effecting change—the three-ring circus. *Am J Health Syst Pharm.* 1999;56:2235-41.

7. Nimmo CM, Holland RW. Transitions in pharmacy practice, part 4: can a leopard change its spots? *Am J Health Syst Pharm.* 1999;56:2458-62.

8. Nimmo CM, Holland RW. Transitions in pharmacy practice, part 5: walking the tightrope of change. *Am J Health Syst Pharm.* 2000;57:64-72.

9. Bloom BS, ed. *Taxonomy of Educational Objectives Book 1: Cognitive Domain.* White Plains, NY: Longman, Inc.; 1984.

10. Krathwohl DR, Bloom BS, Masia BB. *Taxonomy of Educational Objectives; the Classification of Educational Goals, Handbook II: Affective Domain.* White Plains, NY: Longman Inc.; 1964.

11. Simpson EJ. The classification of educational objectives in the psychomotor domain. In: *The Psychomotor Domain, 9.* Washington, DC: Gryphon House; 1972.

12. Festinger LA. *Theory of Cognitive Dissonance.* Evanston, IL: Row, Peterson and Company; 1957.

13. Rogers EM. *Diffusion of Innovations.* 4th ed. New York, NY: The Free Press; 1995.

14. Hepler CD, Strand LM. Opportunities and responsibilities in pharmaceutical care. *Am J Hosp Pharm.* 1990;47(March):533-43.

15. Gottfredson GD. Career stability and redirection in adulthood. *J Appl Psych.* 1977;62(4):436-45.

16. Holland JL. *Making Vocational Choices: A Theory of Vocational Personalities and Work Environments.* 3rd ed. Odessa, FL: Psychological Assessment Resources, Inc.; 1997.

17. Kacmar KM, Carlson DS. Antecedents and consequences of organizational commitment: a comparison of two scales. *Educational and Psychological Measurement.* 2000;59(6):976-94.

Chapter 6
EDUCATION AND TRAINING FOR PATIENT CARE

Christine M. Nimmo, Ross W. Holland, & John P. Rovers

At the 2000 meeting of the Australian Institute of Pharmacy Management, the keynote speaker was Tom O'Toole, an unusual choice for a pharmacy meeting. O'Toole owns a bakery and has no particular expertise in health care.

O'Toole has turned his bakery in Beechworth, a small town in rural Australia, into a multimillion dollar business. This amazing success is not because his cakes are necessarily better than anyone else's or his prices lower. Instead, he is a strong advocate of extensive staff training to support first-class customer service.

After O'Toole's speech, a pharmacist in the audience raised his hand. "Why spend all that money on training?" he asked. "Staff tend to leave after a while, and then you've invested all this money on training them for nothing."

"Yes, that's a worry," O'Toole replied. "But you know what would be worse? Suppose I didn't train them and they stayed!"

He brought the house down.

The next story is apocryphal and concerns two professors, one an older woman with decades of teaching experience, the other a junior faculty member still learning the ropes. One day, the senior professor bet her young colleague $100 that she could teach her dog French within a month. Thinking it a sure bet, the younger woman eagerly accepted. A month went by and the time came to examine the results of the lessons. Upon being commanded to speak French, the dog simply replied "woof."

"You owe me a hundred dollars!" exclaimed the younger professor.

"Not so fast," came the reply. "I just said I was going to teach him French. I didn't promise that he was actually going to learn it!"

These stories illustrate issues and assumptions that will shape the rest of this chapter and that are echoed repeatedly in pharmacies everywhere. Unlike the baker

---

The publisher wishes to acknowledge the American Society of Health-System Pharmacists for the contribution of this chapter, © American Society of Health-System Pharmacists, Inc.

in the first story, all too often pharmacy managers pay little attention to staff training and development. True, some clinical or administrative staff are offered training to support institutional missions, but these efforts do not trickle down to staff pharmacists. If they do, rarely is the training aimed at accomplishing specific goals or objectives. Any positive change that occurs is a wonderful surprise, but likely did not happen by design.

In the community pharmacy setting, the situation is probably worse. Sometimes owners and managers attend continuing education (CE) programs and perhaps they pay staff pharmacists' registration for one local conference per year, but often the only reason pharmacists take part in professional development is to earn enough CE credits to renew their licenses.

Unfortunately, organizations that devote time and resources to staff training and development often find themselves in the position of the young professor, who assumed that being taught (that is, attending the conference) is the same as learning (that is, obtaining the knowledge, skills, and attitudes to do something with the information). Usually, they are just as chagrined when nothing much happens.

This chapter discusses how to create and deliver good learning programs and highlights problems to be aware of when scrutinizing existing programs. It also gives information about organizations that provide pharmaceutical care training materials. Overall, this chapter helps you select from the dozens of CE programs, short courses, home study, and other training options available today and guides you through the steps of creating in-house programs to suit your staff's specific educational needs. Although we often refer specifically to pharmacists, this chapter's advice can be applied to technicians as well.

Planning Your Pharmaceutical Care Training Program

Professional competence is the sum of a pharmacist's skills, professional socialization, and judgment, as Chapter 5 points out. Thus, your training program must address all three of these factors. Although most available programs cover some of these areas, they ignore other vital parts of the competency equation. Some teach pharmacists what to do but do not show them how, or they train in the "what" and "how" but do not explain "why." And most programs do not last long enough for pharmacists to develop much judgment about the skills and knowledge they have acquired. If nothing else, these concerns underscore the need for pharmacy managers to choose wisely from available options. Table 6-1 summarizes some of the published literature that describes pharmaceutical care training programs. The sidebar on page 127 discusses common limitations of such literature.

Table 6-1. Summary of Literature Describing Pharmaceutical Care Training Programs

Author(s)	Program Description	Program Outcome	Comments
Kimberlin et al.[1]	Randomized, controlled study comparing effects of training vs. controls on community pharmacists' patient care activities. Training consisted of prereading and a 1-day workshop.	Intervention group pharmacists were significantly more likely to discuss new medications, ask about problems, provide enough time for patient questions, and provide written information. There were no differences between groups in patient knowledge of medications, compliance, or incidence of drug therapy problems.	Educational program was not well described. Significant outcome measurements are more closely related to traditional patient counseling than pharmaceutical care. System changes in pharmacies not addressed.
Robertson et al.[2]	Descriptive paper on BS-trained hospital pharmacists who shadow clinicians, attend rounds, and discuss and present patient cases.	Pharmacists improved on posttest, increased number and complexity of interventions, increased cost savings.	Very brief description of program, no statistics on outcomes. Practice skills emphasized are more closely related to traditional clinical pharmacy than pharmaceutical care. No control group. System changes in pharmacies not addressed.
Barnette et al.[3]	Descriptive paper of two programs involving community pharmacists. First included readings on hypertension, three workshops on hypertension,	First program's graduates "successfully implemented" the program into practice.	First program includes steps involved in designing a clinical skills program and relevant learning outcomes.

continued on page 123

Table 6-1. Summary of Literature, continued

Author(s)	Program Description	Program Outcome	Comments
Barnette et al.[3], continued	patient care skills, and blood pressure monitoring, and clinical experience in a pharmacist-run blood pressure clinic. Second program describes BS-trained community and ambulatory pharmacists who completed 4-week mini-residency in university teaching hospital. Participants chose from several areas of concentration.	Second program's graduates have developed patient care protocols, asthma care program, brown bag program.	Poor description of outcomes. Physical and systems changes in practice site are not well described. No control group. System changes in pharmacies not addressed. Second program includes good description of educational content. Poor description of outcomes. No control group. System changes in pharmacies not addressed.
Currie et al.[4]	Randomized, controlled study of BS-trained community pharmacists. Intervention group pharmacists received 40 hours training in pharmaceutical care philosophy and practice, patient care skills, and pharmacy and systems redesign.	1,078 patients enrolled over 6 months. Patients of intervention group pharmacists were 7 times more likely to have a drug therapy problem identified, 8 times more likely to receive an intervention by the pharmacist.	Only small number of pharmacists included. Difficulty in recruiting and retaining patients into intervention group. No therapeutics taught to intervention group.
Peterson et al.[5]	Descriptive paper on clinical skills development program in hospital. Part 1: consulting, adverse reactions, documentation, monitoring, medication errors,	Pharmacists rated program highly. Pharmacist interventions increased in areas included in the program.	How education was delivered is not described. Not all skills taught are clearly related to pharmaceutical care. No patient outcomes

continued on page 124

Table 6-1. Summary of Literature, continued

Author(s)	Program Description	Program Outcome	Comments
Peterson et al.[5] continued	drug information, drug interactions. Part 2: variety of therapeutic topics.		described. System changes in pharmacies not addressed.
Grainger-Rousseau et al.[6]	Open, uncontrolled study on developing a practice model to provide therapeutic outcomes monitoring to asthmatics in community pharmacies. Training included asthma management protocols, self-study readings on drugs and asthma, and creating a patient care system.	Pharmacists found capable of providing patient care. Patients, physicians, pharmacists viewed program positively but small numbers of patients actually enrolled. Authors viewed program as a technical success but a marketing failure.	Article describes the assumptions underlying what education should support, but does not actually describe content of educational materials. Educational program said to be published elsewhere, but does not appear to have been published.
Mehra and Wuller[7]	Descriptive paper on series of six workshops (Principles of Pharmaceutical Care; Communications; Documentation, Monitoring, Reimbursement; Clinical Skills in Diabetes, Hypertension, Asthma) plus practicum to develop patient care skills in college preceptors.	Pharmacists' knowledge and confidence in patient care skills and readiness to precept students all improved. Pharmacists made changes in daily practice, provided more patient education, and increased their motivation to counsel patients.	All outcomes are self-reported by pharmacists. Significance of improvements not addressed. Link between improved practice and student precepting not clearly made. No control group. System changes in pharmacies not addressed.
Bennett[8]	Descriptive paper on developing pharmaceutical care certificate program. Home study, work-	Author's observations are that pharmacists have become proficient in using program's components.	Excellent description of educational program. Would be useful in developing

continued on page 125

Table 6-1. Summary of Literature, continued

Author(s)	Program Description	Program Outcome	Comments
Bennett[8] continued	shops, and practice application exercises developed in practice re-engineering, pharmaceutical care practice, disease management, marketing, and reimbursement.		other programs. Very little outcome data presented.
Hagel et al.[9]	Descriptive paper. 5-day workshop over 16 weeks. Conversion program focuses on pharmaceutical care practice skills, site redesign, staff training, marketing, and reimbursement. Program also used college faculty as mentors and several work-group meetings were held with peer pharmacists.	Suggests a positive impact on pharmacists, students, colleges, and practice associations.	Excellent description of educational program. Would be useful in developing other programs. Very little outcome data presented.
Farris et al.[10] and Kassam et al.[11]	Open, uncontrolled study in two related articles describing thought processes, educational program, and outcomes of program in which community pharmacists provide direct patient care. Educational program consists of live programming, self-study, faculty mentoring, and	Trend towards improvement in pharmacist's management of drug therapy problems, therapeutic thought processes, identification of drug therapy problems, and documentation noted, but did not reach statistical significance. Detailed	Excellent description of educational program. Would be useful in developing other programs. Level of detail is considerable and may give impression that the program is too complex to be implemented by others.

continued on page 126

Table 6-1. Summary of Literature, continued

Author(s)	Program Description	Program Outcome	Comments
Farris et al.[10] and Kassam,[11] continued	pharmacy redesign.	results are published separately.[12,13]	
Patterson[14]	Controlled study describing content and evaluation of a year-long certificate program in pharmaceutical care taught via distance learning. Program content included pharmaceutical care skills and therapeutic topics.	Self-evaluations by pharmacists indicated improved knowledge and confidence in patient care skills. Significant improvements in test scores in specific therapeutic modules. Significant improvements seen in several problem-solving abilities. There was a trend for intervention pharmacists to be more likely to interview patients and identify and document problems.	Excellent description of educational program. Would be useful in developing other programs. Small sample size may obscure results.
Reutzel et al.[15] and Reutzel et al.[16]	Descriptive study of developing and evaluating year-long pharmaceutical care skills program for chain pharmacists. Program included self-study plus live programming in communications, patient care skills, and therapeutic topics.	Outcomes were evaluated using focus groups. Participants stated program increased self-confidence and knowledge and was superior to written CE. Time constraints were cited as major limitation. Authors did not observe changes in practice resulting from the program.	First paper describes in detail a wide variety of useful ideas in developing in-house CE. Second paper describes educational program, although only in limited detail.

Pharmaceutical Care Training in the Literature

Reviewing the literature is likely to convince you to create your own educational program, or at least modify an existing one, if you want to transform your practice. Among the problems you're likely to find:

+ Programs with a patient care focus may not reflect true pharmaceutical care or are only useful as part of a pharmaceutical care practice. An example is programs that train staff pharmacists to become better patient counselors.

+ Training programs on therapeutics topics assume that increasing pharmacists' knowledge base will naturally result in practice changes and improved patient care. Although a keen understanding of therapeutics (among other topics) is certainly necessary to provide high-quality pharmaceutical care, you can't assume that increased therapeutics training will, by itself, have a significant effect on outcomes.

+ Literature that outlines how an educational program was developed, though practical and helpful for developing other programs, often lacks an evaluation of the program carried out. In other words, it may look like a good program, but there is no evidence to suggest that it works.

+ Some articles, though they give a thorough evaluation, fail to describe the educational details of a program. Others describe programs in such detail and provide so much practice theory that only the most dedicated managers could possibly slog through them to create useful programs.

+ The literature tends to focus on patient care skills while putting little emphasis on pharmacy systems. Patient care skills are certainly vital, but they don't exist in a vacuum. Both pharmacists and their workplaces need to change.

Understanding Training Principles

If you have a substantial training budget and at least one staff member responsible for pharmacists' professional development and training, you'll find the material in this section useful for creating in-house training programs. For greater detail than is provided here, see the comprehensive guidebook *Staff Development for Pharmacy Practice*.[17] If you're without generous resources—like most managers—this section equips you with an understanding of staff development principles to apply in building a useful training program from in-house materials, conferences, and possibly hired consultants. Overall, this section helps you develop or purchase training programs wisely.

Our discussion is based on the Practice Change Model (PCM) described in Chapter 5, in which pharmacists go through four stages of readiness to learn about practice change. In the first stage, pharmacists find out about the new practice model but do not plan to make changes. In the second and third stages they learn more about the new practice and start trying it out, but have not yet successfully adopted the new practice model. By the end of stage 4, the pharmacists are saying, "I want to do this, I believe I can do this, and I have a plan to get there." They have adopted the values and attitudes of the target pharmacists and are eager to learn.

The optimum time to begin training is when pharmacists are somewhere in the fourth stage. To bring them completely through stage 4, you must assess their ability to perform the desired tasks and then rectify any deficits you find. In this chapter, as we explain the various steps in planning a training program, we're assuming that you have the mindset of a professional trainer. Although it may be the first time you are learning this material, we want to lead you through the process in its ideal form.

The learning resources component of the PCM (Figure 5-4, page 104) suggests that to provide a successful program you need:

+ Resources that match the learners' needs.
+ An awareness that these resources exist.
+ Resources that are accessible.
+ Resources that are affordable.
+ Time to learn.

Matching Learning Needs

Step 1: Analyze Required Knowledge, Skills, and Abilities
You must be able to articulate the practice change you seek for each pharmacist and be sure that each job description states in observable, measurable terms the new tasks to be performed. If descriptions are imprecise, vague, or incomplete—failing to delineate each task in detail—you will not be able to assess pharmacists' present capabilities. Thus you will incorrectly diagnose what they need to learn and you will not develop efficient training tools.

To create job descriptions that are effective guides for staff training, you must analyze each job responsibility and detail the associated tasks. Each job responsibility statement should be discrete and not overlap with other responsibilities. The list of tasks under each responsibility should represent everything the pharmacist must do to fulfill the job responsibility.

Most likely, current job descriptions for your staff lack sufficient detail for you to perform this analysis. The Pharmacy Practice Activity Classification,[18]developed in 1998 by a group of national pharmacy organizations and published by the American Pharmaceutical Association, is a helpful resource for creating job descriptions suitable for task analysis. It breaks pharmacists' job responsibilities into four major domains, each of which has a series of classes of job responsibility. Each class has a number of specific activities, and each activity in turn includes a number of job tasks. Some job tasks are further broken down into individual steps. The book *Staff Development for Pharmacy Practice* can also help you create job descriptions suitable for task analysis.[17] The examples of job responsibilities and tasks below, taken from these two sources, are for a pharmacist who provides medication-use education.

Sample Job Responsibilities and Tasks

Example 1

Domain: Ensuring appropriate pharmacotherapy
Class: Ensure patient's understanding and adherence to his or her treatment plan
Activity: Interview patient
Task: Educate patient/family/caregiver
Activities:

Provide accurate oral and/or written information as appropriate for the patient's treatment plan.

Use visual aids and/or demonstrations.

Demonstrate assembly and use of administration devices.

Discuss use or avoidance of pharmacotherapy.

Discuss use or avoidance of complementary and alternative treatments.

Discuss use or avoidance of nondrug therapy.

Source: *Pharmacy Practice Activity Classification*. Washington, DC: American Pharmaceutical Association; 1998:6.

Example 2

Job Responsibility: Provide medication-use education to patients and caregivers.
Task 1: Design medication-use education for patients and caregivers that effectively meets their needs.
Task 2: Use effective patient education techniques to provide counseling to patients and caregivers, including information on medication therapy, adverse effects, compliance, appropriate use, handling, and medication administration.

Source: Nimmo CM. *Staff Development for Pharmacy Practice*. Bethesda, MD: American Society of Health-System Pharmacists; 2000:76-7.

No matter what source you use to create or modify your pharmacists' job descriptions, you must be sure that each task is worded so that it is observable and measurable, thus providing the statements of performance you need to assess competence.

Step 2: Analyze Capability to Perform Desired Tasks

With an accurate job description in hand, you are now ready to ask "Does the pharmacist already know how to do the new tasks?" If the answer is yes, no training is needed. If it's no, you have some work ahead.

Initially, your analysis will focus mostly on the skills component of the three aspects of professional competence (skills, professional socialization, and judgment) discussed in Chapter 5 (see Figure 5-1, page 96). Pharmacists' capabilities can't be assessed until they are working at Stage 4 and have the required attitudes and values—the ingredients of professional socialization. And they can't develop judgment without extensive practice, so it makes sense to look at skills alone at this point.

Let's say that the pharmacist's job description contains this new responsibility: "to modify or design, develop, monitor, and evaluate patient-specific pharmacist care plans." A new task you have said the pharmacist will have to perform is to "collect and organize all patient-specific information needed to prevent, detect, and resolve medication-related problems and to make appropriate medication therapy recommendations."

How do you tell whether your pharmacist can perform this task successfully? The most practical and potentially accurate method is to ask the pharmacist to create an information base for a real patient and then evaluate the information base against objective criteria. Among criteria appropriate for judging the quality of the information base:

- All necessary information is included: demographic, medical, medication therapy, behavioral/lifestyle, social/economic, and administrative (such as physician/prescriber information, informed consent, and pharmacy policies and procedures).
- No extraneous information is included.
- Sources of information are the most reliable available.
- Information is recorded in a way that facilitates subsequent problem-solving and decision-making.

For each item you should be able to say "yes" or "no," never "partially." The totality of your answers should help you arrive at a summary judgment on task performance. Right now the pharmacist either is or is not capable of performing this task independently in the work environment.

Using direct observation to assess competence is not effective unless you use objective criteria as the standard for measurement. The chapter entitled "Identifying Essential Job Responsibilities" in the book *Staff Development for Pharmacy Practice*[17] provides sets of criteria for most tasks performed in the general practice of pharmacy. Unfortunately, the Pharmacy Practice Activity Classification[18] does not provide these criteria.

Step 2 produces a list of desired tasks that, at the moment, the pharmacist is unable to perform. In other words, it allows you to diagnose what the pharmacist can and cannot do in the new practice.

Step 3: Share the Results with the Practitioner

Now is the time to give the pharmacist an accurate picture of the tasks he or she must learn to perform in the new practice model. Remember that this information is crucial in Stage 4, Making Sure It Sticks (described in Chapter 5, page 112), in which the pharmacist embraces the values and attitudes associated with the new practice. Practitioners need to understand how much effort it will take to insert new professional values into an existing value system so they know how the balance of priorities in their present value system will be affected. If they commit to the new practice based on unrealistic assumptions of what it involves, the commitment may not stick when honoring it steals more than expected from other high-priority commitments in their life.

Step 4: Specify What Needs to Be Learned

In this step you figure out exactly what the pharmacist needs to learn to perform the new tasks. Then you record your conclusions in a way that helps you identify existing training materials or design your own, so you can deliver suitable training.

Imagine that you have evaluated a pharmacist's ability to perform the series of tasks specified for the job responsibility "modify or design, recommend, monitor, and evaluate patient-specific pharmacist care plans." The task statement in the pharmacist's job description reads, "modify or design an evidence-based monitoring plan for a therapeutic regimen so that achievement of patient-specific goals can be effectively evaluated."

You've already assessed the pharmacist's present skills. You had asked him to create monitoring plans for two patients, and neither met the criteria for an acceptable monitoring plan. Your first question is, "What do I suppose that he would need to know or be able to do in order to design a good monitoring plan—limited to things that I don't think he already knows?" Each answer is an instructional objective (IO)— something you need to teach and that the pharmacist needs to learn. As you read through the following list, don't worry yet about the words in parentheses. Focus instead on how to tease out all the things a person who is already a pharmacist might need to learn to prepare a good monitoring plan.

+ IO 1: (Comprehension) Explain the importance of considering what is feasible and useful when designing a monitoring plan.
+ IO 2: (Comprehension) Compare and contrast methods for monitoring patient adherence (e.g., refill rates, questioning, return demonstration).
+ IO 3: (Analysis) Determine monitoring parameters that will measure achievement of goals for a therapeutic regimen.
+ IO 3.1: (Knowledge) State customary monitoring parameters for medical regimens commonly prescribed.
+ IO 3.2: (Comprehension) Explain the relationship between what are normal value ranges for parameters and the influence on those ranges by a given disease state.
+ IO 4: (Analysis) Identify the most reliable sources of data for measuring the selected parameters.
+ IO 5: (Synthesis) Define the desirable value range for each selected parameter taking into account patient-specific information.
+ IO 6: (Comprehension) Explain social issues that should be considered when designing a monitoring plan.
+ IO 7: (Comprehension) Explain factors that should influence the frequency and timing of parameter measurements in monitoring plans.
+ IO 8: (Comprehension) Explain effective approaches to assuring patient returns for follow-up visits in the ambulatory setting.
+ IO 9: (Analysis) Identify the most appropriate person to collect monitoring data (e.g., family member, nurse, patient).
+ IO 10: (Comprehension) Explain the use of treatment guidelines in the design of monitoring plans.

This list identifies 10 things you think the pharmacist must learn in order to do this task. The words in parentheses refer to cognitive learning or problem-solving skills that are used when designing or modifying a monitoring plan. This type of learning is different from the affective learning involved in changing values and attitudes, as discussed in Chapter 5. It is also different from learning psychomotor skills, such as how to insert a needle into an IV bag without destroying the bag.

Figure 6-1, based on Bloom's Taxonomy of the Cognitive Domain,[19] shows the stages of learning that the words in parentheses represent. Learners move from the bottom of the chart—*knowledge,* or regurgitation of memorized information—to *comprehension,* in which they can articulate the meaning of what has been memorized. It is only in the next level, *application,* that learners are capable of actually doing something with what they have learned. The subsequent levels of learning involve more advanced levels of "doing" and higher levels of thinking. From the ability to analyze, learners move to creating new ideas and, at the highest level, making judgments.

Figure 6-1. Bloom's Taxonomy of the Cognitive Domain Applied to Pharmacy Example

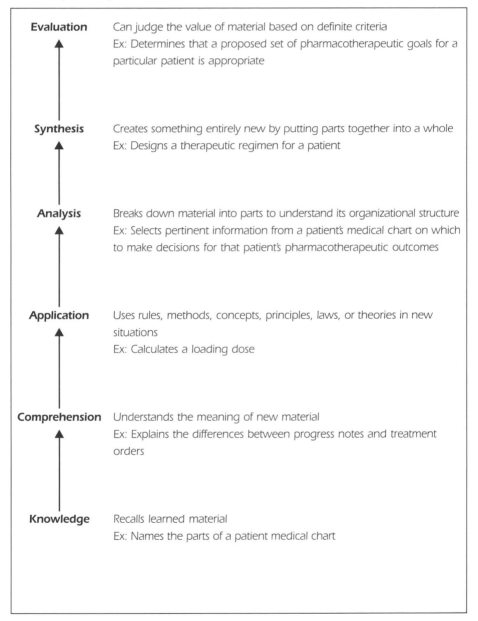

Evaluation — Can judge the value of material based on definite criteria
Ex: Determines that a proposed set of pharmacotherapeutic goals for a particular patient is appropriate

Synthesis — Creates something entirely new by putting parts together into a whole
Ex: Designs a therapeutic regimen for a patient

Analysis — Breaks down material into parts to understand its organizational structure
Ex: Selects pertinent information from a patient's medical chart on which to make decisions for that patient's pharmacotherapeutic outcomes

Application — Uses rules, methods, concepts, principles, laws, or theories in new situations
Ex: Calculates a loading dose

Comprehension — Understands the meaning of new material
Ex: Explains the differences between progress notes and treatment orders

Knowledge — Recalls learned material
Ex: Names the parts of a patient medical chart

Each objective's wording is carefully crafted to describe an observable, measurable behavior that reflects evidence of learning at the specified level. When writing objectives, you must match carefully the verbs you choose and the classification. People who can *explain* something are demonstrating comprehension. Being able to *state* something suggests memorization—learning strictly on the knowledge level.

When you have finished doing a learning analysis for each task you've targeted for training, you will have the entire list of what must be taught. Each task statement tells you what the endpoint of successful training will be.

Rather than performing learning analyses yourself, you can use professional, off-the-shelf sources for most work that pharmacy practitioners perform. The American Society of Health-System Pharmacists has developed standards for general pharmacy practice and for common specialty areas, which can be downloaded off the Web at http://www.ashp.org/public/rtp/.

Step 5: Evaluate the Match of Instructional Resources with Needs

Your list of what the pharmacist needs to learn (the observable, measurable task statements) and the instructional objectives associated with each task tell you what the pharmacist's training must encompass. Let's say you're a professional trainer designing a program for a pharmacist who needs to learn how to create care plans and deliver care to patients with diabetes. Figure 6-2 provides a flow diagram of the tasks involved in developing patient-specific care plans and delivering care for any disease state. You've evaluated the pharmacist's skill in the entire sequence of tasks needed to fulfill this job responsibility and you found that she can do some of the tasks well. Her strengths lie in identifying medication therapy problems, modifying or designing a therapeutic regimen once the goals are determined, and recommending the regimen and monitoring plan so that they are accepted. But she is weak in other areas, which means she can't take a patient with diabetes through all the required steps. Specifically, she has trouble with:

+ Collecting and organizing all patient-specific information the pharmacist needs to prevent, detect, and resolve medication-related problems and making appropriate medication-therapy recommendations for patients with diabetes.
+ Specifying therapeutic goals for a diabetes patient so that they incorporate principles of evidence-based medicine and integrate patient-specific data, disease and medication-specific information, ethics, and quality-of-life considerations.
+ Modifying or designing an evidence-based plan to monitor the therapeutic regimen of a diabetes patient so pharmacists can tell whether patient-specific goals are met.

You are likely to conclude that:

✦ The job responsibility that is this pharmacist's goal involves highly complex intellectual problem-solving.
✦ Achieving the goal depends on the pharmacist stringing together a series of tasks, each involving an intellectual problem-solving skill and each dependent on the other. Consequently, it isn't enough to work on improving the task areas in which she is weak. At some point in her training she must be challenged to put them all together in a smooth flow, as shown in Figure 6-2.

Figure 6-2. Flow of Decisions to Modify or Design, Recommend, Monitor, and Evaluate Patient-Specific Pharmacist Care Plans

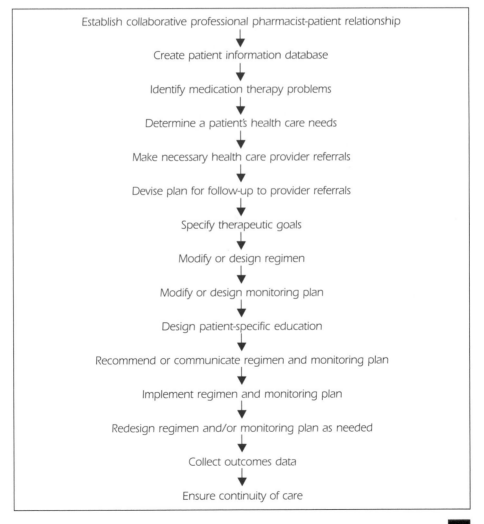

✦ Instruction won't be complete until the pharmacist has actually practiced all the tasks involved in designing and delivering care to diabetes patients and can carry them out with real patients without coaching from the instructor.

✦ Because the learning analysis yielded instructional objectives at many different levels of learning, the most efficient instruction is going to be a mix of methods.

Levels of Learning

The second and third columns of Table 6-2 reveal the appropriate methods for achieving instructional objectives at different levels of Bloom's Taxonomy. You know that achieving any of the objectives classified at the knowledge level, pure memorization, can be done by reading or lecture because memorization does not require interaction with an instructor. But when the necessary learning moves to comprehension and beyond, interaction with an instructor is essential. The two instructional objectives below call for guided discussion (instructor poses carefully framed questions) or interactive lecture (a lecture interspersed with periods of guided discussion).

✦ (Comprehension) Explain the mechanism of action, pharmacokinetics, pharmacodynamics, pharmacoeconomics, usual regimen (dose, schedule, duration, form, route, and method of administration), indications, contraindications, interactions, adverse reactions, and therapeutics for medications used to treat patients with diabetes.

✦ (Comprehension) Explain how other health care professionals' goals influence the therapeutic goals you set for patients with diabetes.

Table 6-2. Methods of Instruction Matched to Bloom's Taxonomy and the Learning Pyramid

STAGES OF LEARNING IN THE FRAMEWORK OF INSTRUCTIONAL STRATEGIES	BLOOM'S LEVELS OF COGNITIVE LEARNING	APPROPRIATE INSTRUCTIONAL METHODS
Foundation knowledge and skills	Knowledge	Reading Lecture
	Comprehension	Guided discussion Interactive lecture
Practical application	Application	Case presentation Case-based teaching Simulation/role play Practice-based teaching
	Analysis	
	Synthesis	
Culminating integration	Evaluation	

According to Table 6-2, four instructional methods are the best choices for the four higher levels of cognitive learning (application, analysis, synthesis, and evaluation). The first, case presentation, requires instructors to reveal the thought process behind each critical decision made to resolve a case. In case-based teaching, the second of the four instructional methods, the instructor presents a case and poses skillful questions. The pharmacist-learner must make and justify each critical decision required to solve it.

Simulation and role play, which together make up the third method, are particularly useful for teaching communications skills. The fourth method is practice-based teaching, or one-on-one clinical teaching by a preceptor. The principles of practice-based instruction—the ultimate method for teaching clinical problem-solving—is illustrated in the learning pyramid in Figure 6-3.

Figure 6-3. The Learning Pyramid

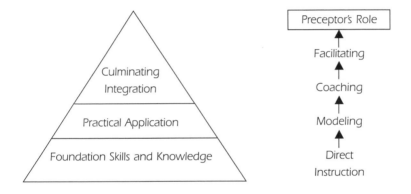

The triangle depicts the progress of learners acquiring an intellectual problem-solving skill, such as the ability to modify or design, recommend, monitor, and evaluate a pharmacist care plan for a diabetes patient. First, learners must acquire basic knowledge and skills about diabetes and its treatment. Next, they must try solving diabetes problems until finally they can put the thinking tasks together smoothly and independently to resolve medication-related problems in diabetes patients. If you look again at Table 6-2, the first and second columns show how the stages in the learning pyramid correspond with the levels of cognitive learning in Bloom's Taxonomy.

Figure 6-3 also indicates the preceptor's role as the learner moves up the learning pyramid. In the first stage the preceptor helps the learner acquire knowledge from content matter: "Read this, attend that lecture, let's discuss," and so on. After the learner understands the material and is ready to try solving a problem, the preceptor should model the thought process involved. For example, the preceptor might do a "live" case presentation in which she talks about a patient case as she solves it: "The lab values seem a little low. Let's see, they've been that way for the last three weeks. Hmmm, it was three weeks ago that we stopped the other medication. I need to do a check in the literature to see if there's an interaction between the two medications . . . ."

After the learner has a model of the problem-solving process to emulate, the preceptor reverts to a coach. As the learner works on a diabetic's case the preceptor asks questions to guide the thought process and provide a stream of feedback. As the learner gets better at solving cases, the preceptor reduces the feedback until the learner is finally ready to tackle a case alone. The preceptor identifies cases at the appropriate level of difficulty and sends the learner off to solve them with the reassurance that the preceptor will be available as needed.

If, like a professional trainer, you know what must be learned and which methods are appropriate for each level of learning, you will search for existing resources that match your pharmacist-learner's needs. (The end of this chapter describes resources that have been developed to help practitioners make the transition to pharmaceutical care.)

You must evaluate each resource against the learning outcomes you have specified to determine whether their instruction method is appropriate. By comparing the wording of your instructional objectives with each program's content description and teaching methodology, you can judge whether a program offers what you're seeking. You know, for example, that a lecture program promising to teach participants how to design therapeutic regimens for diabetes patients really can't fulfill its promise. Despite what the program objectives say, straight lectures provide only knowledge-level instruction.

Modeling and Coaching

When learners are nearly ready to apply foundation knowledge and skills, you need to model for them the thought processes involved in problem-solving. A good approach is to pull out an old case and talk through the way it was resolved, allowing learners to ask questions throughout. It's also helpful for learners to work with a preceptor on real cases so they're exposed to the thought process as it occurs and can experience serendipity's value in problem-solving.

Case-based teaching is useful during the beginning stages of coaching. Some existing training programs use this approach for groups, which is excellent for getting started. Eventually, however, pharmacist-learners must move to a one-on-one coaching situation because in real life they need to rely on their own judgment. Over time, the cases used for coaching should reflect the full spectrum of ages, clinical conditions, and severity that pharmacists must deal with in actual practice.

Preceptors

Cases that learners handle during their first solo flights should be carefully chosen to fall well within their skill level. Bolstering learners' confidence is more important at this point than stretching the limits of their skills.

Any pharmacist-learner who will be providing pharmaceutical care needs an in-house preceptor. In addition to the preceptor's guidance, learners need instructional material—a mix of existing programs and those you create yourself—as well as live continuing education programming with students and the instructor in the same room. We cannot envision teaching pharmacists on your staff how to give direct patient care without including guided experience in your setting with your sources of information, your structure, and your patients.

In some practices, the need for an in-house preceptor is a barrier. What if you don't have anyone capable of filling this role? Alternatives include hiring an outside consultant to provide training, which may, of course, be expensive. Another option is to partner with your local college of pharmacy, which may be willing to provide a faculty member to help with coaching and modeling in return for your pharmacy's participation as a training site for students.

Selecting Resources

Step 6: Be Sure the Pharmacist-Learner Knows the Options

Your training plan will work best if learners help select the learning resources. Because they are the ones who have to use them, they know which ones match their skills and preferences. Your job is to provide full information on the alternatives. If they receive information on the advantages and disadvantages of each program, they are more likely to choose training that they'll want to participate in.

Pinpointing Accessible Resources

Step 7: Determine Timing and Geographic Accessibility

When you consider existing learning resources you must think about where they are offered, when they take place, and how long they take. Perfect programs are no good if they require travel your budget doesn't cover, are at the wrong time, or necessitate days away from the job that can't be accommodated. To avoid missing excellent learning opportunities, try to develop an adequate training budget and plan for substitute pharmacists when necessary.

Assessing Affordability

Step 8: Determine the Cost of Training

Some pharmacies train on a shoestring—combining ingenuity, in-house teaching, and freebies that happen to match learning needs. Others invest considerable money in training. Once you have a reasonable training plan you can compute the budget, considering both obvious and hidden costs, such as:

+ Instructional materials.
+ Registration for continuing education programs.
+ Loss of opportunity costs when diverting in-house staff from regular activities to teaching or developing instructional materials.
+ Travel for training delivered away from the pharmacy.
+ Hiring of temporary or permanent staff to deliver instruction.
+ Temporary staffing to free pharmacists' time for learning.

Step 9: Determine Availability of Training Funds

You need to secure funds to pay for any training necessary to bring about desired changes in the pharmacy's practice. If you're lucky, a foundation or company may be willing to sponsor your program. More likely, however, you'll have to redirect funds from an existing budget line. (To justify a budget for training use the same technique described in Chapter 4, page 77, for justifying your technology budget.) Your business plan, which you learn how to create in Chapter 7, may need to include funding to cover training expenses.

Step 10: Complete the Training Plan

It takes time to resolve the details of a training plan. For the best use of funds, wait until the plan has been written and evaluated for its effectiveness and efficiency to start spending money on training. Even if you choose to outsource all training, you must base that decision on a logical process that includes determining learners' needs and carefully selecting training resources. Following a written plan prevents you from overlooking key details and helps you monitor the program as you go.

Step 11: Secure a Commitment to Pay

Sometimes management decides that pharmacists should pay some or all of their training costs. This is most likely to happen when practitioners pursue a nontraditional PharmD degree to gain pharmaceutical care skills. Paying one's own fees may also be required when pharmacists seek new skills that are above and beyond their job's immediate demands. Even if your pharmacists are not pursuing a major credential like a PharmD, remind them that they are developing skills they can use throughout their career. Paying some of the training cost is not unreasonable because their new skills will make them more marketable. You could also pay for the training but agree that pharmacists who leave your employment before 2 years will reimburse a portion of the cost. The main point is that it's okay to ask pharmacists to pay for part of their training, but not to present them with a training bill if they don't know it's coming.

Addressing Time Issues

Step 12: Create Time for Training

Finding the time for training is a huge issue, both for the learner and the trainer. Among ways to make time available are to change staffing patterns, increase the use of technicians, and bring new technology into the pharmacy, such as dispensing automation. For more discussion of this issue, see Chapter 4.

Step 13: Make Time to Learn

If the change in practice involves significant new learning, it is likely that pharmacists will have to use both free time and work time for training and study. Or, at the very least, they must think creatively about how to make time in the workplace for what they need to learn. Either way, it's important that your pharmacists have a realistic picture of the time and effort needed and believe their efforts will be worth it. Thus, if they are not already in Stage 4, making sure it sticks (see Chapter 5, page 112), you must move them there. Sacrificing their free time or reshuffling their priorities will be more acceptable to pharmacists who have internalized the attitudes and values of the new practice. Other important points to keep in mind:

+ Include pharmacists in the design of training so their preferences are accommodated as much as possible.
+ Restructure the environment as best you can to create the time for training and learning.
+ Don't make unfounded assumptions about slack in your pharmacists' workday. Get into the pharmacy for a reality check.
+ Brainstorm with your pharmacists about ways to create free time.

Doing Things Right

Figure 6-4 is a sort of "crib sheet" to keep you on track as you follow the 13 steps we've described for designing and delivering effective training. Before you jump into the process, however, make sure that education can solve your problems in creating a new practice. If the real barrier isn't your pharmacists' knowledge, skills, and attitudes, but instead it's the system they work in, additional staff development won't help much.

Figure 6-4. Training for Practical Change

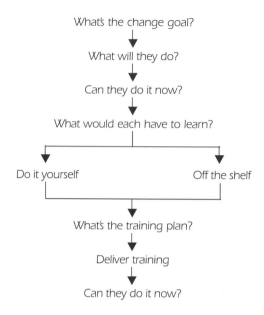

What's the change goal?

What will they do?

Can they do it now?

What would each have to learn?

Do it yourself   Off the shelf

What's the training plan?

Deliver training

Can they do it now?

For instance, if the physicians in your hospital object to pharmacists interviewing their patients, teaching interviewing skills is not the solution. Or if your goal is to convince third-party payers to pay for cognitive services, teaching care plan development will not result in the desired change. All necessary changes in the system must be identified and addressed before you move ahead with education.

You probably never thought that a managerial position would feel a bit like being academic dean of a pharmacy school. But like it or not, changing to the kind of practice that results in safer and more effective medication use requires you to orchestrate practitioners' retraining. To meet this challenge, the best thing you can do is to adopt the mindset of a professional trainer and move systematically through the process this chapter describes.

Available Programs

Because patient care training programs are always being developed and revised, the information below may go out of date quickly. And the fees associated with them are subject to change (which is why none are listed). Before you buy any materials, review your training needs carefully and consider how programs may require modification to fit the particular requirements of your practice.

American Pharmaceutical Association (APhA)
www.aphanet.org

APhA provides a wide variety of certificate training programs for pharmacists who want a more patient-focused practice. Most combine self-study and live programming and offer up to 28 hours of continuing pharmacy education.

You may be able to obtain APhA's original program, "Positioning Your Practice for Pharmaceutical Care: An Individualized Blueprint for Change," through state pharmacy associations partnering with APhA to make the program available. Participants get hands-on training in general patient care and learn how to re-engineer their practices to provide pharmaceutical care including redesigning their pharmacies, creating the time for patient care, seeking reimbursement, and marketing.

APhA also provides disease-management certificate programs, which blend self-study with practice skills, in such areas as asthma, diabetes, dyslipidemias, and immunizations.

American Society of Health-System Pharmacists (ASHP)
www.ashp.org

ASHP offers tools, textbooks, and reference materials for pharmacists changing their practices. It also offers two self-study clinical skills programs that provide a useful foundation for patient care. Targeted primarily at health-system pharmacists, each series contains several modules. The Pharmacotherapy series helps practitioners learn how to review medical charts, create a pharmacist's database, devise a drug therapy problem list, and develop and monitor a pharmacist's care plan. The Drug Information series contains supportive material to help pharmacists analyze a drug information request, retrieve and evaluate drug literature, and formulate a response. Although these are not necessarily direct patient care skills, they do provide useful foundation skills for pharmaceutical care.

Among ASHP's self-study courses for pharmacists in ambulatory settings is the Ambulatory Clinical Skills Program, which provides guidance for collecting and organizing patient-specific information and developing and managing a care plan. Separate programs provide ambulatory care pharmacists with patient care skills both generally and for specific diseases, including diabetes and asthma. All of ASHP's modules carry 2 to 6 hours of continuing education credit.

National Community Pharmacists Association (NCPA)
www.ncpanet.org

NCPA offers a 2-day live program through its National Institute for Pharmacist Care Outcomes (NIPCO) that awards pharmacists a certificate in general patient care skills. Using a mix of didactic lecturing and skill building exercises the program covers interviewing patients, identifying drug therapy problems, developing care plans, and marketing. Among special features are sessions on physical assessment and completing various billing forms. The program carries 20 hours of continuing education credit.

NIPCO also offers 2-day live programs on disease-specific topics including arthritis, cardiovascular disease, diabetes, immunizations, osteoporosis, and respiratory conditions. Each carries 12 to 20 hours of continuing education credit.

American College of Clinical Pharmacy (ACCP)
www.accp.com

ACCP's prime offering for pharmacists seeking patient care training is the self-study Pharmacotherapy Self-Assessment Program (PSAP), which emphasizes an in-depth knowledge of recent trends in drug therapy. Although not marketed towards any specific segment of the profession, this comprehensive, rigorous program assumes that you already have significant underlying knowledge of both pathophysiology and pharmacotherapy. Each of the approximately 12 modules discusses a specific organ system or patient population and carries 10 to 20 hours of continuing education credit.

State and Local Resources

Both state and local practice associations as well as colleges of pharmacy offer a wide range of training. Increasingly, colleges and state associations are partnering to train pharmacists who in turn serve as preceptors for pharmacy students on clinical rotation. Such training tends to be high quality and low cost. One such program is the Iowa Center for Pharmaceutical Care (ICPC), a partnership between the Iowa Pharmacy Association and the Colleges of Pharmacy at Drake University and the University of Iowa. (For details, see http://www.iarx.org.) ICPC offers a combined self-study and live continuing education program for both community and health-system pharmacists moving to a patient care focused practice. This program includes hands-on training, but it is less about teaching specific practice skills than it is on getting pharmacists to think about the type of practice they wish to implement and providing resources for further study. It carries 28 hours of continuing education credit. ICPC faculty also offer site-specific consultation for an extra charge.

References
1. Kimberlin CL, Berardo DH, Pedergast JF, et al. Effects of an education program for community pharmacists on detecting drug related problems in elderly patients. *Med Care.* 1993;31:451-68.

2. Robertson KE, Hultgren SJ, Rhodes RH. Staff development program for identifying and resolving drug therapy problems. *Am J Health Sys Pharm.* 1996;53:2194-6.

3. Barnette DJ, Murphy CM, Carter BL. Clinical skill development for community pharmacists. *J Am Pharm Assoc.* 1996;NS36:573-80.

4. Currie JD, Chrischilles EA, Kuehl AK, et al. Effect of a training program on community pharmacists' detection of and intervention in drug therapy problems. *J Am Pharm Assoc.* 1997;NS37:182-91.

5. Peterson AM, Chase SL. Enhancing pharmaceutical care through ongoing staff development programs. *Hosp Pharm.* 1997;32:361-6.

6. Grainger-Rousseau TJ, Miralles MA, Hepler CD, et al. Therapeutic outcomes monitoring: application of pharmaceutical care guidelines to community pharmacy. *J Am Pharm Assoc.* 1997;NS37:647-61.

7. Mehra IV, Wuller CA. Evaluation of a pilot clinical skills workshop series for community pharmacists. *Am J Pharm Ed.* 1998;62:136-41.

8. Bennett RW. Components of a pharmaceutical care certificate program. *J Am Pharm Assoc.* 1998;38:76-81.

9. Hagel HP, Rovers JP, Currie JD, et al. The Iowa Center for Pharmaceutical Care: an effective education-practice partnership. *J Pharm Teach.* 1998;6(3):19-37.

10. Farris KB, Kassam R, Cox CE, et al. Evaluation of a practice enhancement program to implement pharmaceutical care. *Am J Pharm Ed.* 1999;63:277-84.

11. Kassam R, Farris KB, Cox CE. Tools used to help community pharmacists implement comprehensive pharmaceutical care. *J Am Pharm Assoc.* 1999;39:843-56.

12. Kassam R, Farris KB, Bruback L. Pharmaceutical care research and education project: pharmacists' interventions. *J Am Pharm Assoc.* 2001;41:401-10.

13. Volume CI, Farris KB, Kassam R, et al. Pharmaceutical care research and education project. *J Am Pharm Assoc.* 2001;41:411-20.

14. Patterson BD. Distance education in a rural state: assessing change in pharmacy practice as a result of a pharmaceutical care certificate program. *Am J Pharm Ed.* 1999;63:56-63.

15. Reutzel TJ, DerFalco PG, Hogan M, et al. Evaluation of a pharmaceutical care education series for chain pharmacists using the focus group method. *J Am Pharm Assoc.* 1999;39:226-34.

16. Reutzel TJ, Hogan M, Kazerooni PV. Development of a patient-based practice model in community pharmacy practice: academic practice interface. *Am J Pharm Ed.* 1999;63:119-26.

17. Nimmo CM, Guerreo RM, Greene SA, et al., eds. *Staff Development for Pharmacy Practice.* Bethesda, MD: American Society of Health-System Pharmacists; 2000.

18. *Pharmacy Practice Activity Classification.* Washington, DC: American Pharmaceutical Association; 1998.

19. Bloom BS, ed. *Taxonomy of Education Objectives Book 1: Cognitive Domain.* White Plains, NY: Longman, Inc; 1984.

Chapter 7

CREATING A BUSINESS PLAN FOR PATIENT CARE

Charles R. Phillips & Lon N. Larson

*"Most people are aiming at nothing ...
and hitting it with remarkable accuracy."*

Will Rogers

Because of the nature of pharmacy education and the amount of therapeutic and pharmacological information in the college curricula, most pharmacists receive little or no training in business issues. Yet, as pharmacists strive to enhance their role in the health care system by launching new patient services, they often find themselves needing direction in how to justify their programs. This justification invariably needs to be presented in a business format to administrators, partners, and financiers. Therefore, the goal of this chapter is to explain the importance of a solid business plan and help you identify and implement the plan for successfully expanding your practice. This chapter also provides the basic tools for "selling" your ideas to others.

Chapter 7 is geared towards implementing services rather than products. Services differ from products in a variety of ways and, as a result, are marketed differently from traditional pharmacy products.[1] Although other books have been written on preparing business plans and even on the individual components of a plan,[2,3] this chapter gives you a straightforward, condensed roadmap for creating a business plan for patient-centered services.

Finally, this chapter provides useable and application-based information for pharmacists in retail and institutional settings. By providing you with examples and cases, you can easily develop a sound plan of action for implementing patient-focused pharmacy services.

Throughout the chapter, you will read about a common case in which a cholesterol monitoring program for at-risk patients is implemented. The case involves Clinic Pharmacy, a small pharmacy located in a medical clinic. Many of the issues of the case cross practice settings and are applicable to independent, large and small chain, clinic, and inpatient pharmacy settings.

Importance of the Business Plan

Planning and formulating a business plan is essential to the growth of a business. Because the business plan is so important, it needs to be created by one or more insiders who know the pharmacy and its patients—not by an outside, hired consultant. Most often, this insider will be you—the pharmacy owner/manager. Likewise, in the institutional setting, the plan should be created by one or more people who know the pharmacy department and the workings of the institution—most often the pharmacy director.

Creating a business plan forces you to organize and prioritize ideas. In times of low reimbursements and staffing, it is imperative that you pursue only the ideas with the best chances for success. The business plan forces you to take an objective look at your pharmacy before embarking on expanded patient services. This ultimately will prevent you from implementing a program without addressing the many details that could make or break the new service.

The marketing component of the plan also helps avoid the all-too-common phenomenon of "if we build it, they will come." Just because a pharmacy has an interest or specialty in a certain program or disease state doesn't mean patients have a need for it. The marketing section of the plan, in particular, bridges the gap between patient needs and pharmacy activities.

The business plan serves two more important functions.[2] When finalized, it becomes the roadmap for implementing the new services and ideas. Without the plan, it becomes far too easy to skip the equally important business details and jump ahead to patient care. After all, it is our nature to focus on patients rather than business.

The business plan also communicates your ideas to other stakeholders outside the pharmacy. The plan communicates ideas in a standard, organized manner that is identifiable to stakeholders like hospital administrators, potential coworkers, health care professionals, suppliers, and financiers. Thus, the business plan becomes the tool to allow others to buy into and support the pharmacy's planned expansion.

Before you begin, there are a few important characteristics of a good business plan you should consider. First, your business plan needs to be flexible and dynamic. A good plan of action compensates for changes in the pharmacy, economic, or political environments. As a result, you should construct the plan in a way that allows for changes in personnel, financing, or institutional support.

Second, your business plan must contain an evaluation component. This will enable you and any stakeholders to determine whether the plan has been implemented correctly and, more importantly, if the plan is reaching the desired outcomes. Without measurable outcomes, you will have no way to demonstrate that your new service is having positive effects. Examples of measurable outcomes can include anything from improved satisfaction or quality of life for patients, to increased job satisfaction for pharmacists, to increased profits for the business. For more on outcomes, see Chapter 9.

Components of the Business Plan

Although different people set up business plans in slightly different ways, most plans have common elements that form the basis for clearly representing the business idea.[2,3] This chapter touches on the 10 elements of a business plan. Because some of these elements are either self explanatory or dependent on the specifics of each pharmacy, some are explained in less detail than others. In addition, some elements, such as financial data analysis, are explained in Chapter 8.

Business Plan Element #1: The Executive Summary

The executive summary is a one- to two-page synopsis of the entire plan. In medical terms, it is the equivalent of the abstract for a journal article. The executive summary succinctly tells the readers the highlights of the business plan and gives them a broad, general understanding of the project before they read the details of the plan.

The executive summary sets the tone for the plan. If it is well written and organized, it gives the impression that the entire project is equally well thought out and appropriate. On the other hand, if the summary is disjointed and incomplete, readers may be left with the impression that the idea is also ill conceived and poorly planned. Therefore, the executive summary must give readers a positive impression of the project to gain their support and interest in pursuing the plan.

Business Plan Element #2: Description of the Business

To begin the process of business planning, it helps to lay the groundwork for the people involved. In the case of a business plan, laying the groundwork includes describing the current business situation. This description provides a frame of reference for the reader to understand the environment and the amount of work and change that will be necessary for the project to succeed.

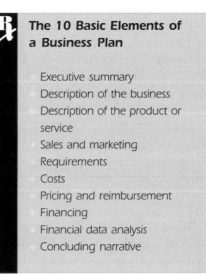

The 10 Basic Elements of a Business Plan

Executive summary
Description of the business
Description of the product or service
Sales and marketing
Requirements
Costs
Pricing and reimbursement
Financing
Financial data analysis
Concluding narrative

You should include a description of the physical layout and assets of the pharmacy in this section. Where is the pharmacy located? What is the staffing situation? What is the history of the pharmacy and its employees? What are the current products, services, and activities the pharmacy offers? By answering all these questions, you will give the reader a perspective on what is needed to successfully deliver the service. Is there a need for employees with different skills? Will the pharmacy need to be moved or reconfigured? Based on history, will the staff and patients accept and use the new services?

CASE EXAMPLE:
Description of the Business

Clinic Pharmacy is a retail pharmacy located in a family practice clinic. The clinic includes 15 physicians and 5 physician assistants, and has a patient base of approximately 200 patient visits per day. The clinic staff is made up of 6 general practitioners, 3 pediatricians, 3 obstetricians, 1 gastroenterologist, and 2 endocrinologists. Clinic Pharmacy occupies 400 square feet of office space in the clinic and fills 180 prescriptions per day. There are 1.5 FTE pharmacists and 1 FTE technician for the pharmacy. The pharmacy is open Monday through Friday, 9 am to 5:30 pm.

Although this description gives a good "physical" portrayal of Clinic Pharmacy, it does not include information such as the services already being offered, amount of spare room in the pharmacy, current skills of employees and their acceptance of change, economic status of the patients, and patients' ability or willingness to pay for services.

These factors should be easily quantifiable in terms of full-time equivalents (FTEs), square footage of space, and employee credentials. But this section also needs a narrative to make the descriptions more real and applicable to what you require. For example, you can describe employees in terms of FTEs to assess personnel costs, but what about their character, work ethic, and commitment? Are they up to a new challenge? Do they have the skills necessary for the new business endeavor? Will they seek out new job skills? Will they encourage or hinder change in the pharmacy? These humanistic ideas are often more important than looking solely at how many bodies are available for working on the project.

Business Plan Element #3: Description of the Product or Service

In this section, you should present readers with a clear description of the new service. This description should outline who has an interest or role in the project (stakeholders) and clearly describe what will be done, how it will be done, and who will do it. Make sure you describe all aspects of the project, from actually performing the service to supporting it and measuring its success.

Business Plan Element #4: Sales and Marketing

Perhaps the most valuable component of a business plan is the marketing section. This section identifies a demand for the service and the method of presenting it to patients. The marketing section becomes especially important when discussing a service like pharmaceutical care. While many pharmacists and pharmacy managers/directors are comfortable with the idea of marketing a traditional *product* such as a prescription, they know much less about the marketing strategies and patient perceptions of a new *service*.

Like the overall business plan, the marketing component helps identify the important issues and potential obstacles in implementing pharmacy care services. This section also helps set a course of action for implementing and evaluating the marketing efforts. The marketing plan can be developed in different ways, but most plans have common features.[4] These features include:

+ Micro and macro environmental analysis.
+ Projected demand and sales.
+ Analysis of competitors.
+ Marketing objectives and strategies.
+ Action plans.

By addressing these issues, the plan shows financiers, partners, administrators, and other stakeholders that you have addressed the most essential aspects of implementing the program—identifying a demand for the service and how to present it to the public. Although this is not an exhaustive list of what can go into the marketing section of a business plan, these five areas provide a firm foundation for successfully launching new services. In addition, they provide a logical order that will help you move the plan along.

 CASE EXAMPLE: Describing the Product or Service

Clinic Pharmacy will implement a lipid screening and monitoring program for patients at risk for coronary complications. This program will include identifying patients at risk, contacting patients, and setting up appointments. At the initial appointment, a staff pharmacist trained in the lipid profile procedure will take patient histories. The pharmacist will also use a finger stick blood sample to obtain a complete lipid profile from a Cholestec LDX analyzer. The pharmacist will then perform a risk assessment, counsel the patient, and schedule follow-up meetings.

To enhance this description, other information should include how you will identify the "at risk" patients, how documentation will occur, and what method you will use to inform prescribers of the service.

For instance, the environmental analysis is a logical starting point to determine what a pharmacy's strengths and weaknesses are, but it also looks at any opportunities and threats. As a result, you can begin to explore whether or not your proposed service has a place in the market. This naturally leads to analyzing projected demand for the service and potential competitors. Once you determine that there is a market for the patient service, you can set objectives, devise strategies, and make plans to actually implement the program.

Environmental Analysis

An objective review of the environment is one of the best tools you can use for making decisions. To be useful, the review must look at what is happening in the pharmacy setting and its immediate surroundings (microanalysis), as well as what is happening within the pharmacy profession and the economy as a whole (macroanalysis). After reviewing these factors, you can develop a clearer plan of action.

A commonly used technique for performing these environmental reviews is called "SWOT" analysis—the critical review of the strengths, weaknesses, opportunities, and threats of the pharmacy's micro and macro operating environments. (See Chapter 1 for a discussion of SWOT analysis applied to planning for patient care.) Quite simply, the SWOT analysis helps identify the strengths possessed, the opportunities to seize, the weaknesses that need improvement, and the issues and groups that could threaten the success of the service.

When performing the SWOT analysis, you can identify internal strengths and weaknesses by asking questions such as:

+ Do we have the resources to conceive, produce, promote, and distribute our services?
+ Do we have or can we obtain financing for the project?
+ Is there someone in place who can manage and implement the new services?

Similarly, examples of questions for identifying external opportunities and threats include:

+ What is the political climate of the profession and our work setting?
+ Are potential customers and other stakeholders receptive to the idea?
+ Is technology or expertise available for such an endeavor?
+ Is there a suitable or potential market for these services?
+ Is adequate reimbursement possible?
+ Do competitors exist in this market or do other people offer similar or substitute services that would be more attractive than ours?

✦ Are there certification or other legal requirements that we must meet before implementing patient services?

By identifying these issues, the manager can focus on the strengths of the pharmacy's staff and business and look at where to best use those talents.

Demand

One of the most common mistakes individuals make when they have a new idea is to ignore what the public really needs, wants, or desires. Often, a business creates a product or idea and then tries to create demand for that product. Although this may be successful if there is a latent demand, it's better and safer to find out what the public wants, and then create and adapt products, services, and business strengths to meet these needs. This point cannot be over-stressed. There must be a perceived or real need for the services being implemented. Otherwise, no amount of expertise or desire will enable the new program to succeed.

Gauging the demand for new services is never easy, but there are ways to esti-mate potential demand. You can query patients and prescribers on whether they

CASE EXAMPLE: SWOT Analysis

Strengths: Clinic Pharmacy maintains good relationships with physicians and other prescribers. We can easily remodel the pharmacy office space into a testing and monitoring area. We have well-trained and enthusiastic staff who are eager to implement these services.

Weaknesses: Clinic Pharmacy lacks reimbursement from insurers. We have not quantified demand in our clinic area. Finding free time to monitor patients and the program, in light of current prescription load, is questionable.

Opportunities: We can identify potential "at risk" patients and monitor other patients more closely. The program can help Clinic Pharmacy increase revenues. Pharmacists may attain professional growth. The pharmacy manager has a special interest in lipid management.

Threats: Clinic prescribers may not support the program or may feel threatened. Clinic prescribers may already be monitoring patients very closely.

Additional questions you should raise in a SWOT analysis include:

   Is there time to manage the program and adequately promote it?
   What financial reserves are available for the project?
   Is the prescription business solid enough to survive without new services?
   Can we alter workflow or use robotics to free pharmacist time?

would use or recommend the services. Unfortunately, this method is time consuming and can also produce answers that are biased. Depending on how you pose the question, people may provide the answer they think you desire.

Alternatively, you can assess the demand at other pharmacies offering a similar service. However, if only one pharmacy in a given area is implementing patient-specific services, it will be impossible to gauge demand in the immediate area. In this case, you will have to estimate demand based on similar programs that others have implemented around the country.

A third option is to make good-faith estimates based on the pharmacy's patient demographics. For example, if a pharmacist believes she can best specialize in a particular disease state, she can easily use her computer system to determine how many patients have diseases such as asthma, diabetes, coagulation disorders, or hyperlipidemias. Similarly, institutional pharmacies can look at the types of specialty clinics and prescribers at their facilities to determine if they have access to a particular patient population.

**CASE EXAMPLE:
Projecting Demand**

Clinic Pharmacy will identify patients based on prescription use for hypertension, hyperlipidemias, and diabetes. Based on published data from pharmacy journals, we expect to enroll X percent of these "at risk" patients in the monitoring program.

Examples of other information you should include in demand projections are:

Types of physicians and patients in the clinic.
Patient load at the clinic.
Physician acceptance/buy-in of your program.

Competition

Who is the competition? This question should be asked in conjunction with determining the demand for a new service or program. In the institutional setting, competition may come from physicians, nurses, or other health care workers who may be offering patient-centered services that affect medication management. In the retail setting, there may be other pharmacists offering similar services. Likewise, many clinics and physician offices may already offer services that pharmacists are now implementing.

In addition to business competitors, you should consider political and inter-profession opposition. For example, many times pharmacists who start programs such as lipid screenings, coagulation clinics, and bone density screenings are challenged by other health care professionals or their state associations. Therefore, the pharmacy should challenge itself to identify potential competition and opposition and address the concerns of these groups. Often, you can preempt opposition when others realize that all parties involved can thrive as public and patient awareness builds for these services.

Marketing Objectives and Strategies

Like any business endeavor, you need a clear action plan for implementing patient services. First, you should state the key objectives for marketing your services. Good marketing objectives should have a time component and be measurable. This means that your objectives will need to have an implementation deadline and a process for measuring the results. Without clear objectives for marketing the service, it becomes far too easy to spend large amounts of resources on unfocused and ineffective messages.

Your marketing objectives may encompass a wide variety of issues. For example, you may want to focus your objectives on increasing awareness for your services. In this case, your objectives should include promotional strategies such as advertising, personal selling to patients and prescribers, public relations campaigns, and sales campaigns. They can also include educating stakeholders about the services and their effects, and enhancing the pharmacy's image. Or perhaps you need marketing objectives to reduce resistance to your new program. If so, your objectives would include ways to create referral systems from prescribers or to inform the public, payers, and health care providers about the benefits of your new service.

Once you have your objectives written, you need to address what marketing tools you will use to meet your objectives. These tools are your marketing strategies. Here, you should address issues such as the 5 P's of marketing and other basic marketing ideas, including:

**℞ CASE EXAMPLE:
Marketing Objectives
and Strategies**

Clinic Pharmacy will implement a lipid screening and monitoring program by January 1st. We will make all potential customers currently patronizing Clinic Pharmacy and all clinic physicians aware of the program via mailings or personal contacts prior to implementation. We will enroll 150 patients by the end of the first year of operation (roughly three patients per week). We will attain a 95% retention rate (patients staying in the program after the initial week).

Examples of other information you should include in your marketing objectives and strategies are:

- **What pricing strategy do you want to follow?**
- **What is the bottom line objective?**
- **How many physicians will refer patients by year's end?**

+ What services do the patients need (product)?
+ Who will you target with these services and what ideas are being presented to the patient (position)?
+ What price will you charge for the services (price)?
+ How will you promote the services (promotion)?
+ Where and how will the services be performed (place)?

Again, stating these issues will help you clarify them for the pharmacist, as well as for the people who will provide support or approval for the project.

Action Plans

Finally, your marketing plan—like your business plan—should have clearly developed action statements. Like the marketing objectives, these statements should have time constraints and be explicit. They should state what will be done, when it will be done, who will do it, and how much it will cost. It is especially important that you include detailed action plans for promotion to both patients and prescribers. In addition, there should be an action plan for evaluating the success of the efforts. Did we meet our objectives? If not, what contingency plans do we have in place to either alter our services and efforts, or to reevaluate our objectives?

CASE EXAMPLE:
Action Plans

We will mail a survey to each patient we screen and monitor within two weeks of each visit to determine their satisfaction with the service. One month before implementation, we will develop and order professional brochures and flyers. One week before implementation, pharmacy staff will place flyers for the service throughout the clinic offices. Patient promotion will consist of a personal letter from the pharmacy manager to everyone identified through prescription records. Pharmacy staff will personally talk with these people when they receive prescriptions from the pharmacy and explain health benefits and risk reduction. Two weeks before enrolling patients, the pharmacy manager will describe the scope of the program and the referral process during his or her visits to clinic physicians.

Examples of other information that you should include in your action plan:

When and how will you contact your local prescribers?
When and how will you evaluate success? Profit or loss?
Employee satisfaction? Demand?

Business Plan Element #5: Operating Requirements

This section of the business plan describes what you need to implement and continue the project. Knowing these needs, which are called "operating requirements," helps lay the groundwork for the next section of the business plan. This is an exercise in identifying the resources and quantities you will need for the project, such as personnel, equipment, remodeling needs, training, and marketing requirements. After pinning down these operating requirements you must assign a dollar cost to them. From there, you can calculate the total cost of the project and its breakeven point. In addition, you will gain a clearer understanding of the project's feasibility, given current resources and business structure.[1]

Business Plan Element #6: Costs

To judge the profitability of the new service, you must obtain an accurate accounting of the costs. Cost is defined as the value of the resources used to produce a service or operate a program. Generally, these resources include labor (personnel time), plant (buildings), equipment, and supplies.

There are four classification schemes used to determine or analyze the cost of a service:

+ Total, average, and marginal costs.
+ Variable and fixed costs.
+ Direct and indirect costs.
+ Capital and operating costs.

Total, Average, and Marginal Costs

Total cost is the sum of all resources consumed by a program, including variable, fixed, direct, and indirect costs. Average cost is simply total cost divided by the units produced. Marginal cost is the change in total cost to produce an additional unit. Table 7-1 illustrates the relationships among these three cost definitions.

Generally, the cost of any service follows the pattern shown in Table 7-1, although the specific numbers will be different. The average cost curve is shaped as a "u," with cost on the vertical axis and output on the horizontal. Average cost initially decreases as production increases. This is sometimes referred to as "economies of scale." However, this trend does not go on forever. Eventually, average cost begins to increase. This is also where marginal cost begins to increase. At this point, you have reached capacity and inefficiencies develop. For example, your personnel may have to work overtime at increased wage rates, or you may have to use equipment beyond its capability, which necessitates more repairs. These factors increase your average cost.

Table 7-1. An Illustration of Total, Average, and Marginal Cost

(a) Units	(b) Total Cost	(c) Average Cost	(d) Marginal Cost
10	5,000	500	
20	8,000	400	300
30	9,000	300	100
40	16,000	400	700
50	25,000	500	900

Average Cost: The average cost (c) can be determined by dividing (b) by (a).
Marginal Cost: The marginal cost—the cost associated with producing additional units—is determined by subtracting the units and total cost at the current level of production from the units and total cost in the desired level of production. The difference in cost is then divided by the difference in units to derive the marginal cost. For instance, in the figures above, increasing production from 30 to 40 units (an additional 10 units) is associated with an increase in cost of $7,000 ($16,000 minus $9,000). Thus, the marginal cost of these units is $700 per unit ($7,000 divided by 10 units).

To solve this problem, you can increase capacity, such as personnel or equipment. In the case of Clinic Pharmacy, if the pharmacy manager thought the current staff was at maximum workload, he or she might hire an additional person to help. This would be an example of increasing capacity and costs of the program.

Cost Definitions

Total cost: the sum of all resources consumed by a program, including variable, fixed, direct, indirect, average, and marginal costs.
Average cost: total cost divided by the units produced.
Marginal cost: the change in total cost to produce an additional unit.
Variable costs: costs that change as your level or volume of production changes.
Fixed costs: costs that do not change as your output changes.
Direct costs: resources that are used exclusively in the production of a particular service.
Indirect costs: resources used in the production of several services, commonly referred to as "overhead."
Capital costs: resources that have a useful life of more than one year, such as equipment and machinery.
Operating costs: resources consumed within a year, including the portion of a capital expense used in that year.

Variable and Fixed Costs

As the level or volume of production changes, it is essential that you understand the distinction between variable and fixed costs. Your fixed cost does not change as your output changes. As its label implies, it remains fixed. In contrast, your variable costs do change as your output changes. Let's look at a simplified example.

A child's lemonade stand has these resources: a table, a pitcher, a lemon squeezer, lemons, sugar, and plastic cups. The first three resources are fixed. Whether the child sells one cup or 100, the amount spent on those resources (the table, pitcher, and squeezer) remains constant. Note that the average fixed cost (total fixed cost divided by units produced) decreases as the output increases, but total fixed cost remains the same. The last three resources used in the lemonade stand are variable. As more lemonade is made and sold, the amount spent on these resources increases. As output increases, the total variable cost increases, while average variable cost remains the same (the cost of sugar in the 100th cup is the same as the first, but the total cost of sugar would be 100 times greater).

You need fixed and variable costs to calculate your breakeven point. This is the point where your revenue equals your total cost and you make a profit. Contribution margin—the difference between the price you charge for an item and your variable cost to produce that item—is central to calculating the breakeven point. When total fixed cost is divided by the contribution margin, the quotient is the number of units that must be sold to break even. At the breakeven point, the producer begins to make a profit. The profit from each item sold is the contribution margin.

Now let's apply this to our lemonade stand example. Let's assume that total fixed cost is $10, the variable cost for each glass of lemonade produced is 30¢, and the selling price is 50¢ per glass. From this information, we can calculate the contribution margin and breakeven point. The contribution margin is calculated as 50¢ (selling price) minus 30¢ (variable cost) which equals 20¢. The breakeven point is the total fixed costs divided by the contribution margin ($10 divided by $0.2 = 50 units). Our stand will break even once we sell 50 glasses of lemonade.

Direct and Indirect Costs

Another classification of costs is direct and indirect. Direct costs include those resources that are used exclusively in the production of a service. An indirect cost, on the other hand, is used in the production of several services.

Indirect costs are commonly referred to as overhead. For example, in a hospital pharmacy, the wages of pharmacy personnel are a direct cost of the department, but the cost of hospital administrators, who oversee several departments, are indirect. Similarly, in a community pharmacy that has a prescription department and a "front end," a pharmacist who spends all of his or her time in the prescription department is a direct cost, while the manager who manages the entire pharmacy is an indirect expense.

Indirect costs need to be allocated to each service or line of business. As a rule of thumb, allocating personnel is based on percent of effort, building-related expenses (rent, utilities) are allocated on square footage, and all other expenses are allocated based on sales. This is a very simplified description of allocation. But it can get very complex, especially in large firms like hospitals.

Capital and Operating Costs

A final classification is the distinction between capital and operating costs. Capital costs include resources that have a useful life of more than one year, while operating costs refer to resources consumed within a year. Operating costs are also referred to as recurrent costs, and they may be fixed or variable.

An example of a capital cost is equipment with a useful life of more than a year. The portion of a capital expense used in a particular time period becomes an operating expense for that period. For instance, if a $9000 machine is expected to last 3 years (with no salvage value), an operating cost of $3000 is assigned to each of those 3 years.

Assigning the cost of a capital expense to various time periods can become quite complex. Accountants rely on various methods of calculating depreciation. The example above illustrates simple straight-line depreciation.

Determining the Cost of a Service

Although many nuances exist between individual services and programs, cost determination can be viewed as a three-step process:

1. Identifying resources.
2. Estimating quantities.
3. Assigning dollar values.

Before determining costs, you must prepare a detailed description of what will be done to patients, where, by whom, and how often. This information is essential so that costs can be accurately assigned. Using your description, the first step in determining costs is to identify the resources—people, building, equipment, and supplies—that you need to produce the service. You should be as thorough and comprehensive as possible in generating this list of resources. Label resources as one of three types: capital, operating/fixed, or operating/variable.

Your second step is to estimate the quantity or number of units of each resource you need to produce the service. You can express this figure as hours of pharmacist time, number of monitoring units, supplies needed for each patient, and so on.

The third step in determining costs is to assign a dollar value per unit for each resource (e.g., wage per hour or salary per year). These are the prices that you have to pay to obtain the resources (e.g., local wage rates rather than national rates).

Table 7-2 provides a framework for the data you will need to determine costs. When reviewing this example, here are a few points to keep in mind:

+ Although the list of resources in the left column is not exhaustive, it includes many of the resources commonly used in pharmacy services.
+ As mentioned earlier, capital expenses have useful lives of greater than one year. You can obtain the depreciated value from the accounting department, or as a rough estimate, you can divide the purchase price by the years of useful life for an annual figure (assuming there is no salvage value).
+ Some personnel may be assigned to a program for a specified amount of time— for example, one afternoon a week. In this case, costs are expressed as percent of effort or number of hours. Also, this is a fixed cost that does not vary as the number of patients changes.

Table 7-2. Resources Common to Pharmacy Services

Capital/Start-up		Price
Plant (remodeling)		depreciation per year
Equipment (life > 1 year)		depreciation per year
Fixed (recurrent)	**Units**	**Price**
Personnel (salaried)	% time; hours	salary + benefits per month
Training, CE	# programs	$/program
Certifications/Licenses		$/year
Hepatitis B vaccination		$/year
Hazardous waste disposal		$/year
Rent		$/month
Utilities		$/month
Phone		$/month
Office supplies		$/month
Maintenance agreements		$/year
Marketing (signage, ads, letters, etc.)		$/year
Variable (recurrent)	**Units**	**Price**
Personnel	hours per patient	hourly rate
Patient supplies	1 per patient	$/unit

+ Other personnel may provide services as needed—for example, each time a patient arrives. This is a variable expense that will increase as patients increase. All variable costs should be valued per patient. In this way, you can easily estimate total costs for differing workloads.
+ Finally, many of the building-related costs are priced per month. These costs are fixed.

CASE EXAMPLE: Determining the Cost of a Service

Clinic Pharmacy wants to implement a cholesterol disease management program. The spare area in the pharmacy (80 sq ft) will be furnished with a desk and chairs. The rent and utilities attributed to the program will be based on one-fifth of the pharmacy's annual charges for the space it occupies (80/400 sq ft). For each new patient, the pharmacist performs a drug regimen review (30 minutes) plus initial counseling and a cholesterol level check (30 minutes). The equipment and supplies needed to perform the monitoring include a Cholestec LDX Analyzer, lancets, alcohol wipes, latex gloves, band-aids, LDX test strips, marketing materials, training, hazardous waste disposal, and a waiver to the Clinical Laboratory Improvement Amendments (CLIA) so that blood tests can be legally performed. The pharmacist expects to monitor the patients' lipid levels twice per year. There will be two additional counseling sessions for a total of four visits per year or two hours per patient. Before starting the program, the pharmacist intends to become certified as a cholesterol disease manager ($500 for training and exams). In addition, a library of books and videos was purchased by the pharmacy ($300).

As illustrated in Table 7-3, the total fixed cost for the first year is $5200—the sum of all capital and recurrent costs. This amount will be spent, regardless of the number of patients participating. The variable cost is $84 per patient per year—$60 in personnel costs and $24 in patient supplies.

Let's assume the patient is charged $120 per year for the program (pricing is discussed later in this chapter). With the projected patient load of 150 patients, the total cost of the program during the first year is $17,800—$5200 in fixed costs and $12,600 in variable costs ($84 x 150 patients). Total revenue is $18,000 ($120 x 150 patients). The breakeven point is 144 patients, which is the fixed cost of $5200 divided by the contribution margin of $36 ($120 - $84).

Note that some of these costs can be reduced if assumptions change. For example, if the office space were used for more than one program, then the rental cost would be split between them. The total and fixed costs for the lipid management program would then be reduced—and so would the breakeven point.

Table 7-3. Expenditures for Clinic Pharmacy's Cholesterol Monitoring Program

Capital/Start-up	Purchase Price	Yearly Cost
Plant (remodeling)		
(furnishings)	$500	$100 (5 year life)
Equipment (life > 1 year)		
Cholestec LDX	$1500	$500 (3 year life)
Educational books, video	$300	$150 (2 year life)
Fixed (recurrent)	**Units**	**Price**
Training, CE	1 pharmacist	$500
CLIA waiver		$150/year
Hazardous waste disposal		$300/year
Rent		$2000/year
Utilities		$500/year
Marketing (signs, letters, etc.)		$1000/year
Variable (recurrent)	**Units**	**Price**
Personnel	2 hours/patient/year	$30/hour
Patient supplies	2 lab tests/year	$12/test
(lancets, alcohol wipes,		
gloves, test strips)		

Business Plan Element #7: Pricing and Reimbursement

Pricing patient care services is a complicated undertaking for many reasons. All too often, we forget that consumers do not purchase based solely on price. If they did, surgeries would be performed by the lowest bidder. In reality, consumers purchase for a variety of reasons, including price, perceived quality, loyalty, how comfortable they are making the purchase, and convenience. No matter what the pharmacy setting, deriving a price for the services should be a combination of evaluating costs, competition, and the patient's/payer's willingness to pay.[5]

By following the steps outlined in the previous section on costs, you will be forced to develop realistic costs for your service and will be able to determine whether the service loses money, breaks even, or makes a profit. Although making a profit is preferable, sometimes it is acceptable to break even or even lose some money on the service if other benefits arise. These benefits may include gaining new patients or having patients increase store traffic and make additional purchases. Of course, in the institutional setting there really are no additional impulse purchases. In this case, additional benefits may be limited to increasing patient and staff satisfaction as well as improving patient care and outcomes.

In determining price, a good place to begin is to look at customer willingness to pay and cost—in other words, the situation that would exist if there were no third-party reimbursement. As discussed earlier, services do not necessarily need to make money. Rather, they may accomplish other goals that are worthwhile such as increasing customer loyalty or improving job satisfaction. Nevertheless, assessing cost data is valuable in setting a price.

There are two pricing schemes for services that you may find helpful. One strategy is to set a global charge for all services in the program. For example, you could charge a quarterly or monthly fee that entitles the patient to all of the services included within the program. Another avenue is to charge a fee for each service you provide. In this case, the initial visit would have a fee, as would follow-up visits, monitoring services, and so on. It is important to remember that third-party programs may require fee-for-service pricing. They don't want to pay for services that are never delivered, which may happen when you offer a package of services for a global charge: patients may not show up for each appointment or take advantage of everything the package includes. So if you charge a global fee, you may also need to price the component services.

Because third parties rarely pay for patient care services provided by pharmacists, it is probably a safe assumption that they will not cover your service. One way to get around this is to require payment from the patients and then let them seek payment from their health insurance company. In this case, you can provide documentation in a format the patient can submit to the insurance company for possible reimbursement. This format includes a pharmacist or medical services claim form such as the HCFA 1500 or the NCPA Pharmacist Care Claim Form.[6,7] Supplying this form is also a good way to remind the patient that they received something. The documentation makes the service more tangible.

Business Plan Element #8: Financing

The business plan should contain a section that talks about how you will fund the project. Funding is based on two main sources—internal and external. Internally, funds may be provided by the owner (self or private funding), from the business itself (profits from current business/department), or in some cases, from a parent company or corporation (such as a pharmacy's corporate office or hospital corporation). Externally, funding sources include banks or other financial institutions, outside private investors, and venture capital firms.

Internal and external funding sources are the individuals who will read and evaluate the final business proposal. The quality and breadth of the business plan will directly influence these groups. Although financial analysis is covered in Chapter 8, be sure you integrate it with your business plan. Potential investors will require some form of financial analysis of the proposed project, including a breakeven point and annual net profit.

Business Plan Element #9: Financial Data

When discussing project finances, certain pieces of information become important. First, a historical perspective of the department or business's finances is key. For example, in a hospital setting, a pharmacy director who can show the past financial contributions of his or her department to the hospital's bottom line will be in a strong position to demonstrate that the department can continue to manage projects and services in a profitable manner.

The second piece of information you must provide is a set of pro forma financial statements. These are estimated financial statements for the first 6 months or 1 year of the project's existence. By setting a price and estimating costs and demand, you can create an income statement that shows projected revenue and profits for the operation.

Finally, the plan should provide information on contingencies. What will projected sales and revenues be at different levels of demand? This deviation analysis will show different scenarios of success for the project. For example, what sales do you need to break even? To produce a 15% return on investment?

Business Plan Element #10: Final Narrative

The last component of the business plan summarizes the plan. This section states the conclusions you have developed based on the previous sections and analyses. Much like the conclusion section of a journal article, you should keep the narrative concise and point out the major findings of the plan. In addition, the summary gives you an opportunity to reiterate why you developed the plan—either for internal use or external use, for planning purposes, or for gaining financing from the reader.

Final Thoughts

The preceding discussion covers a large amount of information in a short amount of space. Although the chapter lays out and discusses a comprehensive business plan, the amount of time and effort to complete such a plan remains daunting. Free time in the workplace is increasingly difficult to come by, but the long-term benefits of finding that time and using it to develop a business plan are great. Up-front planning can potentially save you money and many hours of work and frustration.

Using the business plan should be an ongoing endeavor. Revisit and alter the business plan periodically. Through this process, you can monitor the project for success and then make any adjustments to coincide with the changing practice environment.

References

1. Kotler P, Bloom PN. *Marketing Professional Services.* Englewood Cliffs, NJ: Prentice Hall; 1984.
2. Bangs DH. *The Business Planning Guide: Creating a Plan for Success in Your Own Business.* Chicago: Dearborn Financial Publishing, Inc; 1998.
3. O'Hara PD. *The Total Business Plan: How to Write, Rewrite, and Revise.* New York: John Wiley and Sons; 1995.
4. Kotler P. *Marketing Management: Analysis, Planning, Implementation, and Control.* Englewood Cliffs, NJ: Prentice Hall; 1988.
5. Rovers JP, Currie JD, Hagel HP, et al. Reimbursement. In: *A Practical Guide to Pharmaceutical Care.* Washington, DC: American Pharmaceutical Association; 1998:151-66.
6. Poirier S, Buffington DE, Memoli GA. Billing third party payers for pharmaceutical care services. *J Am Pharm Assoc.* 1999;39(1):50-64.
7. Krinsky D. Reimbursement for pharmacist care services, part 2. *America's Pharmacist.* September 1999:47-51.

Chapter 8
FINANCIAL MANAGEMENT FOR PATIENT CARE
John M. Chapman

You may be wondering why there is a chapter on financial management in a book about creating and implementing a patient-centered practice. Somehow, patient-centered services and financial management don't seem like terms that belong in the same sentence. However, if you refer back to Chapter 1, you will recall that you were asked to answer four questions about your practice:

1. Where are you now?
2. Where do you want to be?
3. How will you reach your destination?
4. How will you know when you have arrived?

The primary goal of this chapter is to help you answer question number 4—How will you know when you have arrived? For some readers, this chapter may also be useful in answering question 3, since financial goals are probably part of your practice development plan. But while you are focusing on how to manage your practice to better care for patients, it can become easy to lose track of one other important issue: If you cannot financially sustain patient care, it will be very difficult for you to continue this component of your practice. In other words, if you cannot afford to keep the doors open, the clinical quality of your patient care doesn't matter.

Different readers may use this chapter in different ways. For example, experienced owners may use this chapter as a review of familiar material. They will then need to consider how to apply these ideas to their new practice initiatives. Other managers, including hospital department heads and chain pharmacy managers, may be less familiar with the topics discussed in this chapter. These readers may find it useful to learn how to calculate and track the financial performance of patient care, as well as to determine what that portion of the practice is actually worth. By becoming well informed about the financial issues related to patient care, you will be in a better position to discuss patient care initiatives with your financially oriented superiors. Since senior administrators rarely learn how to speak "clinically," it behooves most clinician-managers to learn how to speak "administratively."

This chapter will discuss two major financial management topics. The first section on financial accounting describes how accountants and others collect and use financial information to calculate how much money a business makes and how much it is worth. Readers can use these concepts to calculate the profitability of their patient care practices. The second section discusses some basic concepts of management accounting. Once you know what your patient care business is worth and how much money it makes or loses, you can use some of these basic management accounting principles to maximize your patient care revenues and minimize costs.

Accounting 101

"Show me the money!" This seems to be the cry from all directions, whether it is the revenue-collecting arm of government, corporate shareholders, your boss, your hospital administrator, your business or domestic partner, and, sometimes, even your children. With all these people looking at a slice of the action, or wanting you to report on what the action is, the question of managing financial information becomes much more pressing.

Every time someone mentions "accounting," most listeners' eyes glaze over and they fall asleep before the first sentence is over. Yet accounting is really only about selecting, collecting, arranging, and reporting the flow of financial information within a business entity. The design of the selecting, arranging, and reporting is usually determined by the needs of the end-user. As a result, the information that you need to manage your business will usually differ from what is required by the government's revenue collection agency or shareholders.

What Is Accounting?

Accounting is selecting, collecting, arranging, and reporting the flow of financial information within a business entity. There are three main types of accounting information:

Management accounting techniques generate the information that helps you run your practice.

Financial accounting techniques provide managers and shareholders or other interested external parties with an idea of the business' worth and profitability.

Tax accounting techniques supply the information needed for tax and regulatory purposes.

All three methods use the same basic information about your business. The only difference is that the data are rearranged into a report format that suits the needs of the specific audience.

There are three main types of accounting information:

+ **Management accounting techniques** generate the information that helps you run your practice.
+ **Financial accounting techniques** provide managers and shareholders or other interested external parties with an idea of the business's worth and profitability.

+ **Tax accounting techniques** supply the information needed for tax and regulatory purposes, according to the legislation and rules governing assessable income and allowable deductions, or by the relevant accounting standards.

All three methods use the same basic information about your business. The only difference is that the data are rearranged into a report format that suits the needs of the specific audience.

This chapter will discuss ideas related to financial and management accounting, but will not cover tax accounting.

Financial Accounting

For most pharmacy operations, "business" is about selling either products or services. Although there are tangible differences between products and services, a key similarity is that no matter which you are selling, you incur costs as you generate sales revenue. Since this book is about providing patient care, this chapter focuses on accounting as it applies to offering a service. The process of financial accounting provides evidence for whether the payments you receive adequately cover your expenses and helps you determine your profit margin.

Selecting and Collecting Financial Data

At its simplest, tracking the flow of money in your practice means recording "money in" (cash receipts) and "money out" (cash payments), and determining the "money left" (profit or loss). This is illustrated in Figure 8-1. You must record all money transactions in an account ledger so you can later create standard accounting reports that show profitability (Profit/Loss Statement) as well as the overall dollar value of the business being conducted (Balance Sheet).

Whether you are tracking the financial performance of a smoking cessation program in a community pharmacy that bills patients individually, or of multiple pharmacist-run ambulatory clinics in an integrated health system that bills several managed care plans, the process for collecting and reporting financial data is the same. Only the amount and complexity of the data will vary. The most important aspect of managing the flow of financial information is to learn what is happening and when it is happening so you can make informed decisions that ultimately improve financial performance.

Figure 8-1. Tracking the Flow of Money

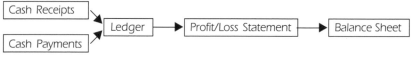

Selecting and collecting the financial data you need to assess your patient care venture should be governed by a few simple accounting rules:

+ **The information must be *relevant* to the issue at hand**. For example, information on revenues generated or costs avoided that you can attribute to specific patient care services can be useful in assisting with managerial decisions. Also, information on the revenue or cost-savings generated by each pharmacist will be valuable when considering productivity. However, the color of the pharmacist's hair is almost certainly not relevant.
+ **The information must be *significant* enough to make a difference in the context in which it is placed**. Once you collect the information, what do you do with it?

How Do You Gain Support for a New Patient Service?

If you practice within a department of a hospital, health system, or managed care environment that focuses on cost containment, your cash receipts are usually minimal or nonexistent. In this case, financial performance is measured against whether you can provide services within your department's allocated budget. The cost of providing your patient service is thus included in the overall budgeted expenses for your department and factored into the entire organization's profit/loss statement and balance sheet. Because you get no direct revenue for the service you must only track expenses associated with providing it and include those data in the department's budget reports.

To gain support for a new patient service, you will need to demonstrate the relationship between the costs your department incurs to provide the service and the costs avoided or reduced in other budget categories. Because you probably don't have direct control over any revenue line in your department, the best way to show efficiency and effectiveness is to compare the year-to-year cost, percentage of sales, or percentage of the department budget. If you can show that spending $x on an initiative has reduced another cost by $x + y, then you have justification for the expenditure that you can use to convince others.

If you work in clinical programs, clinical services, or on formulary committees, you are probably familiar with the concept of incurring a cost to avoid or decrease a larger cost. Examples of these proactive cost-reduction strategies include promoting preferred formulary products, switching patients from parenteral to oral therapy, initiating therapeutic protocols, or making greater use of group purchasing contracts. Table 8-1 illustrates a sample 3-year budget in which the annual dollar allocations to the pharmacy are decreasing, yet the department is still managing to introduce and fund innovative practices. This is because the innovative practices have helped reduce the drug budget and probably helped maintain the other labor costs.

In a pharmacist-run clinic in a health system, all the financial information for the health system is presented in its Annual Report in an aggregated form. Expenses for long-distance telephone calls or copy supplies would not be listed in the Annual Report. Trustees and others do not need to see detail at this level. However, these types of expenses are relevant for management accounting purposes, and will be discussed later in the chapter.

✦ **The information must be *timely* and available to be acted on**. Unless the information is presented at a time when we can use it, it loses much of its value. While it may be somewhat useful to know that the patient care part of the business started to fail 12 months ago as a way of explaining severe financial difficulties now, it would have been much better to see this when it had started and fix it then.

Table 8-1. Three-Year Annual Budget Summary

Year	2000	1999	1998
Budget allocation	$1,640,000	$1,660,000	$1,800,000
Sub-area Costs			
Clinical Programs	$50,000	$25,000	$25,000
Lipid Management Service	$30,000	$0	$0
Other Labor	$60,000	$55,000	$50,000
Drugs & Consumables	$1,500,000	$1,600,000	$1,750,000
Operating Surplus/ (Deficit)	$0	$(20,000)	($25,000)

Arranging Financial Data

Simply put, arranging is grouping "like with like." As shown in Figure 8-2, we group all the cash receipts together and all the cash payments together. Initially, these repetitive items are grouped in the cash receipts and cash payments books. Things such as fees paid by patients, services billed to third-party insurance, and over-the-counter products (OTCs) or patient self-monitoring equipment sold as a direct result of patient services provided are recorded in receipts. Wages, purchases of OTCs and equipment, rent, and so forth are recorded in cash payments.

Groupings in a hospital pharmacy may be very different from those in a community pharmacy. The other thing that you will notice is that there is a column with the heading "Sundries." The reason for this is simple—there will always be some items that won't fit into the major groups. So instead, you simply record them in the sundries column and separate them out in the next stage.

Realistically, most pharmacies will have an automated "point-of-sale" system that records sales transactions in predefined categories. Nevertheless, it is still im-

Figure 8-2. Cash Receipts and Payments

CASH RECEIPTS BOOK							
Date	Description	Bank	Services 3rd Party	Services Cash	Sales OTC	Sales Equip	Sundries
1	Daily Receipts	350		200	150		
2	Daily Receipts	300		100	200		
3	Daily Receipts	460	200	60	200		
4	Daily Receipts	115		40	75		
5	Daily Receipts	380		80	50	250	
6	Daily Receipts	810		60	500	250	
7	Daily Receipts	505		80	425		
8	Daily Receipts	325		120	105	100	
9	Daily Receipts	385		140	45	200	
10	Daily Receipts	350		200	150		
11	Daily Receipts	400		100	300		
12	Daily Receipts	152		120	32		
	TOTALS	4532	200	1300	2232	800	0

CASH PAYMENTS BOOK							
Date	Description	Chk No	Amount	Equipment Purchases	Wages	Rent & Utilities	Sundries
1	All Prop Ltd	251748	140			140	
2	API	251746	800	800			
3	J Smith	251747	389.39		389.39		
4	Cholestech	251745	400	400			
5	D Craig	251749	256.36		256.36		
6	Power Utility	251750	230.32			230.32	
	TOTALS		2216.07	1200	645.75	370.32	0

portant to identify the relevant patient service categories that you will need financial data for and work with the system vendor to ensure cash receipts and payments are captured correctly.

The cash receipts and payments books enable you to record a great deal of useful information, including:

+ The date, the amount of money you banked, and the source of that money.
+ The date, the check number, the amount of the check, and what the payment was for.

In addition, laying this information out in columnar format allows you to *cross check* the addition of the columns, since the total in the "bank" or "amount" columns should equal the sum of the other columns.

If you close books at the end of the month, you will have a monthly summary of the major categories and a collection of the "sundry" items. To group "like with like," the next step is to move or "post" the column totals and individual sundry items from the cash books to the next stage of the aggregation process—the ledger. A ledger account allows you to aggregate both receipts and payments in one place and gives you a net result.

At its simplest, the ledger is nothing more than a series of cards or computer files in which you account for cash in and cash out according to some category, such as wages or a particular third party payer. Although each column in your cash receipts/payments book will most likely have a corresponding ledger account, additional ledger accounts can provide further detail and allow you to track costs for specific business components with greater accuracy.

As cash enters the practice from patients and payers, or leaves the practice for wages, supplies, or other expenses, it is entered into the ledger based upon entries in your cash receipts and payments book. A modified cash payments column and ledger account can also help you track the cost-savings associated with a particular service.

Proprietorship or Owner's Equity

The process of accounting was developed as a way of calculating a person's or a household's worth. To do this, it became necessary to collect and arrange data in a meaningful way so that a person was able to:

+ Estimate their worth (assets).
+ Gain an understanding of what was owed to them and owed by them (liabilities).
+ Determine a net amount (owner's equity).

As illustrated in the equation below, the value of the business or the *owner's equity* is determined by subtracting the liabilities from the assets. The balance is left to the owner.

$P = A - L$ Where P = Proprietorship or the owner's equity in the business
A = Assets of the business
L = Liabilities of the business

Under accounting theory, assets *belong* to the owner and debts are the *responsibility* of the owner. Assets and liabilities are two of the major items on a balance sheet that represent the business's financial position *at a point in time*. On a given date, the balance sheet shows that the practice had assets of $X, liabilities of $Y, and the business was worth $Z.

Conversely, the concepts of revenue and expense are summaries of activity *over a period of time*. Revenue and expense are two of the major items on a profit and loss statement and indicate that over a given period, the business spent $X, collected $Y, and had $Z left over as profit.

Recognizing Revenue and Expense

As previously discussed, revenue and expense are incurred over a period of time. Therefore, you will need to consider at what point to "stop the flow" to evaluate what your revenues and expenses are over some period of time. You can recognize revenue when you:

+ Acquire resources.
+ Receive customer orders.
+ Produce goods and services.
+ Deliver goods and services.
+ Collect cash.

Usually, you recognize revenue in an operating cycle when the following criteria are satisfied:

+ You have performed the principle revenue producing service.
+ You can accurately predict any costs necessary to produce the revenue that you have not yet incurred.
+ You can objectively estimate the amount you will ultimately collect in cash or its equivalent with a small range of error.

Ledger Accounts and Double Entry

Debits and credits are simply names for a side of an account in a ledger, commonly called a *T account*. As shown in Figure 8-3, this is because the layout of the account is in the shape of a T.

Definitions of Common Accounting Terms

Asset—An asset is any future service in money or a future service convertible into money that is legally or equitably secured to some person or set of persons. To be an asset:

+ There must be a future right to a service that must have a positive and non-zero value;
+ The right must be specific; and
+ The right must be legally enforceable.

Liability—Conversely to an asset, a liability is a legally enforceable obligation to a person or persons outside the business entity.

Revenue—Revenue is the monetary expression of the goods and services transferred by an enterprise to its customers over a period of time.

Expense—Similarly to revenue, expenses are also incurred over time. Expense is the cost over a given period of the flow of goods or services into the market and of related operations. An expense can be considered a decrease in net assets for the creation of revenue. The assets used to generate revenue can include cash, equipment, supplies, inventory, or even printed materials used for patient education sessions.

Figure 8-3. Ledger Account Structure

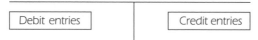

In a typical double-entry bookkeeping system, one side of any accounting transaction must be "posted" to the debit side of the ledger and the other to the credit side. Increases in assets and decreases in liabilities are treated as debits. Liabilities, owner's equity, and decreases in assets are treated as credits.

As shown in Figure 8-4, the first ledger account is for medical equipment and indicates an increase in assets (debit) when cholesterol cassettes were purchased into inventory. A refund for a glucose meter was recorded as a credit since it actually was returned and therefore resulted in a decrease in medical equipment assets.

The related entries for the cash ledger account are opposite. The refund for the glucose meter is shown as a debit since the cash asset has increased, while the payment for the cholesterol cassettes reduces the cash asset.

Figure 8-4. Sample Ledger Accounts

| MEDICAL EQUIPMENT | | | | | | |
Date	Notation	Debit Amount	Date	Notation	Credit Amount
4/10/01	Cholesterol Cassettes	400.00	9/15/01	Glucose Meter	200.00
CASH IN BANK						
Date	Notation	Debit Amount	Date	Notation	Credit Amount
9/15/01	Glucose Meter	200.00	4/10/01	Cholesterol Cassettes	400.00

After posting entries to a ledger account over the course of a time period, you can reach a net result by adding up the debits and credits for each different ledger account. The difference between the debits and credits for each ledger account is then transferred to the Profit and Loss Statement and the Balance Sheet. The Profit and Loss Statement (P/L Statement) shows the business activity in a historical perspective over a period of time. The Balance Sheet shows the activity at a point in time, which is the end of the period of time shown in the Profit and Loss Statement. For example, the P/L Statement may show activity for the period of January 1, 2001 through December 31, 2001, while the Balance Sheet shows activity on December 31, 2001. You can use these reports to evaluate how much money you have made on patient care programs and how much the patient care practice is worth (owner's equity). Figure 8-5 provides a sample P/L Statement and Balance Sheet.

Figure 8-5. Reporting on Financial Information

SAMPLE PROFIT/LOSS STATEMENT FOR XYZ PHARMACY		
For the Financial Year Ending June 30, 200X		
SALES	A	
Less:		
Cost of Sales	B	
GROSS MARGIN	A – B	[1]
Less:		
EXPENSES		
Accounting	C	
Advertising	C	
Bank Charges	C	
Cleaning	C	
Depreciation	C	
Electricity & Services	C	
Freight & Cartage	C	
General Expenses	C	
Insurance	C	
Interest	C	
Motor Expenses	C	
Rent & Outgoings	C	
Salaries & Wages	C	
Total Expenses	Sum C's	[2]
NET PROFIT	[1] – [2]	

BALANCE SHEET FOR XYZ PHARMACY				
As of June 30, 200X				
ASSETS		LIABILITIES		
Current Assets		Current Liabilities		
Cash on Hand	A	Accounts Payable	AA	
Accounts Receivable	B	Cash at Bank	BB	
Cash at Bank	C			
Stock on Hand June 30/0X	D			
Total Current Assets:	Sum [1]	Total Current Liabilities:	Sum [3]	
Noncurrent Assets		Noncurrent Liabilities		
Fixed Deposits	E	Loans	CC	
Goodwill	F			
Total Noncurrent Assets:	Sum [2]	Total Noncurrent Liabilities:	Sum [4]	
		Owner's Equity	[5]	
Total Assets	Sum [1]+[2]	Total Liabilities	Sum[3]+[4]+[5]	

175

Management Accounting

Profit and Loss Statement and Balance Sheet reports generated by financial accounting methods will definitely help you answer questions such as, "Did I make a profit?" or "What are my assets and liabilities?" However, these types of summary documents typically do not provide much information on how these results were achieved and, more importantly, what can be done to manage and improve the process. This is the realm of management accounting.

Management accounting uses exactly the same data as financial accounting. It has to, since the business under consideration is the same. However, management accounting examines and interprets the data differently. Where necessary, it also collects additional material—often nonfinancial in nature—that will improve the interpretation of the data set.

Management accounting looks at information that will help you in your day-to-day role of maximizing revenue and minimizing costs. By understanding what your revenues and costs are, what influences them, and how to maximize revenues and minimize costs, you can create an economically viable patient care practice. Some key management accounting concepts that will help you classify costs and revenues are described below.

Revenue

For purposes of this book, revenue will usually mean sales of individual consultations to patients that are either paid for by the patient or billed to third party payers. But remember, the "items" of revenue will vary as the business varies. For instance, wholesalers or drug companies may be a source of revenue if they have their own programs to subsidize the creation of patient care practices in pharmacies and elsewhere.

Costs

Business costs represent the value of economic resources that are sacrificed to obtain more valuable resources. The common element of costs is that they represent resource transformation—the flow of resources from one form to another. For example, the resource or "cost" of a pharmacist's time can be transformed into revenue (a more valuable resource) when she charges a patient for performing education and drug therapy monitoring as part of an asthma care program.

When categorizing costs, you can group them by:

+ **Natural characteristics,** such as materials, equipment, and labor. In this situation, costs are defined according to their properties. For example, materials are described as materials and labor is included as labor.

+ **Intended function**, such as manufacturing, marketing, and administration. When you group costs this way, you assign them to the part of the operation that incurs them. For example, marketing costs are incurred by the marketing department and may include the labor, materials, rent, advertising, and other costs that the marketing people use to do their work.
+ **Association with a product or service**, such as direct or indirect costs. *Direct costs* are those costs that are clearly attributed to the creation of a product or service. For example, the cost of the cassettes used to perform blood cholesterol monitoring as part of a hyperlipidemia clinic is a direct cost. *Indirect costs* are those costs that cannot be directly attributed toward the creation of a specific product or service, but are still required to run the whole operation. For example, there may be janitorial costs to clean the pharmacy at night, but it becomes difficult to determine just how much is attributable to the lipid clinic unless you are allocating expenses based on the proportion of square footage devoted to patient services.
+ **Tendency to vary with activity level changes**, such as fixed and variable costs. Grouped this way, costs are described as fixed or variable depending on whether the cost varies with changes in input. For example, rent will be a *fixed* cost since the rent will be the same, even if the pharmacy is closed. On the other hand, if you hire an additional part-time pharmacist to help you vaccinate patients during influenza season, you can eliminate the cost of this labor once flu season is over and therefore you would consider it a *variable* cost.

The decision on how to group costs will vary according to the type of information you need to make business decisions. The particular dollar value you assign to a cost can vary, but generally should be the purchase price paid for the resources used. Economists will often use an additional concept of *opportunity cost—the value of alternative resources foregone*. For example, if you spent all your money on a diabetes program, you have foregone the opportunity of investing that same money in the stock market. The lost potential profit would be termed the opportunity cost.

It is important to realize that cost groupings are not necessarily mutually exclusive, and a particular accounting method may require both actual and opportunity costs. Having several descriptors available can be confusing, but ultimately, managers can calculate their costs with greater precision. For instance, your total costs may look acceptable, but perhaps your variable costs for staff training are too high. If you did not calculate your costs in a variety of ways, you would not be aware that this particular type of cost was out of control.

The final issue you must consider when allocating costs is to decide when the cost was incurred. Generally speaking, the costs of providing a patient care service are attached to that service and are incurred when the service is sold. In other words, in your anticoagulation clinic, the cost of the pharmacist's time and the cost for the lab supplies to provide the service are not incurred until the service is actually provided.

Cost and Revenue Allocation

Revenues can be allocated on the basis of product, geography, or both. When allocating revenues, first you must consider whether the center is a:

+ **Cost center**, where only costs are measured; or a
+ **Profit center**, where profit margins are the object of measurement.

To differentiate between a cost center and a profit center, consider the typical hospital pharmacy. The hospital pharmacy provides pharmaceutical products and related services to patients but does not bill patients separately or receive revenue directly. Because patient charges for pharmaceuticals are included on a patient's hospital bill or are covered by prospective payment from a third party, the department would be considered a cost center. The reverse is true for a pharmacy operation that bills patients or third-party payers directly to offset operating expenses and is expected to contribute any profits to the organization's overall financial picture.

Categorizing Costs

When categorizing costs, you can group them by:

- **Natural characteristics**, such as materials, equipment, and labor.
- **Intended function**, such as manufacturing, marketing, and administration.
- **Association with a product or service**, such as direct or indirect costs.
- **Tendency to vary with activity level changes**, such as fixed and variable costs.

The decision on how to group costs will vary according to the type of information you need to make business decisions. It is important to realize that cost groupings are not necessarily mutually exclusive, and a particular accounting method may require both actual and opportunity costs. The final issue you must consider when allocating costs is to decide when the cost was incurred. Generally speaking, the costs of providing a patient care service are attached to that service and are incurred when the service is sold.

Whether you should consider your patient care practice a cost center or a profit center is especially important to managers practicing in a health-system setting. In this case, you must ensure that your administrators will allow you to allocate your patient care revenues in an advantageous way. In other words, if you believe that your diabetes education program will never turn a profit, considering such revenues as a profit center will most likely result in the program being viewed as a failure. Alternatively, if the program has the capacity to reduce other costs in your department or decrease costs in another department (and hopefully improve patient outcomes as well), then you are well on the way to retaining the service. Remember that the cost-reduction can also take the form of downstream cost-avoidance, such as reduced length of hospital stays, less use of health services, or fewer lost days from work.[1]

Putting It All Together

To illustrate and apply the theory outlined above, it may help to return to the case example from Chapter 7. In this example, Clinic Pharmacy wishes to introduce a lipid screening and monitoring program for at-risk patients.

The costs cited for Clinic Pharmacy have most likely come from the historical financial management accounts prepared by the accountants for the pharmacy, and from records kept by the pharmacy. The costs for expenses such as labor, rent, and office supplies come from these historical accounts or from quotations sought for this purpose if the pharmacy is new to the business. Note also that, in the case of Clinic Pharmacy, some "nonfinancial" information has been included in the calculations, such as the area of the pharmacy that has been set aside for this service. This allows management to estimate the "cost" of rent for that area of the pharmacy taken up by the service, and enables them to calculate the total cost of providing the service. Using what you've just learned about management accounting, you can extend this principle to examine other aspects of the proposed service.

Under the cost and pricing assumptions used in the case example, for 150 patients, the pharmacy will have an operating surplus of $200 in the first year ($18,000 in revenues, less $17,800 in fixed and variable costs). It is important to note how sensitive this surplus is to ways in which you define revenue and cost. If you immediately account for all of the fixed costs, rather than sharing them over the expected life of the project or the expected life of the asset, then you will arrive at a very different—and negative—result.

You can also turn your management accounting focus towards either the revenue or surplus aspects of the service. Assuming that at least some of the space and other resources used for the lipid screening service were already available in the pharmacy, the question from a management view is, "Is this the most productive use of the resources?" The case example notes that the area used for the testing is "spare." But what if this is not the case? What if you have to cease or scale down one activity to make way for another? Then the question becomes which is the most productive activity? Which one generates the greatest surplus? To perform this calculation, you will need to go back and calculate the productivity of the previous activity.

If the previous activity produced a greater operating surplus than the lipid screening service, then a decision to proceed with the lipid screening service may still be made on the basis of patient need or health outcomes. However, the difference between the surplus from the original activity and the lesser surplus from the screening service becomes the *opportunity cost* of proceeding with the less profitable service.

As this discussion illustrates, it is essential for a manger to dissect and manipulate both revenues and costs in this way to gain an understanding of the dynamics of the business rather than a purely historical knowledge of what has gone before.

Benchmarking with Key Performance Indicators

Understanding the dynamics of the business will usually involve the calculation of *key performance indicators* (KPIs), which calculate relationships between different aspects of the financial inputs and outputs, often combined with some other non-financial information, such as size of the pharmacy and number of staff. Some examples include:

+ Sales per square meter or square foot.
+ Sales per dollar of wages paid.
+ Gross profit per square meter or square foot.
+ Net profit per square meter or square foot.
+ Gross margin return on inventory investment (GMROII).
+ Gross profit per lineal meter or foot of shelving.

As you may imagine, you can calculate many different types of relationships and indicators, such as "Prescription revenue per patient over 65 driving 1980 Chevy Corvettes." In order to determine what to calculate, remember the criteria for selecting information that were introduced at the beginning of this chapter. The information and what it will be used for needs to be relevant, significant, and timely. The above example probably fails both the relevance and significance tests.

However, the whole point of calculating KPIs is to compare competing or alternative services in a pharmacy, or performance and efficiency across different pharmacies. In Australia, they use the *Guild Digest*, produced by the Pharmacy Guild of Australia for this purpose. In the United States, the *Searle Digest* performs a virtually identical role. Figure 8-6 gives examples of various benchmarks used in Australia. Although there are no benchmarks for patient care, the patient care services you offer can still impact your pharmacy's performance. For example, by improving customer loyalty and increasing prescription volume after implementing patient centered services, you may positively impact total sales, profit margins, and inventory turnover. This can improve the overall financial performance of the pharmacy.

Figure 8-6. Key Performance Indicators for Advice-Wise Pharmacy

KPIs—Advice-Wise Pharmacy			
Year Ending June 30, 1999			
	1999	**1998**	**Guild Digest 1999**
SALES			
Sales/square meter	**$13,107**	**$11,511**	$10,141
Front Shop Sales/Turnover	**29.32%**	**27.06%**	35.59%
Front Shop GP$/Total GP$	**32.00%**	**28.00%**	N/A
Script Numbers	**62,408 (5%)**	**59,395**	38,155
Script Numbers per Hour	**21.82**	**20.77**	12.88
Average Prescription Value	**$25.24 (5%)**	**$24.03**	$23.80
PROFITABILITY			
Gross Profit	**31.49%**	**32.36%**	32.79%
Operating Profit/Sales	**12.40%**	**11.80%**	3.44%
STAFF			
Wages/Sales	**10.02%**	**10.85%**	11.00%
Sales per Hours Opened	**$779**	**$684**	$475
EXPENSES			
Rent/Sales	**2.42%**	**2.75%**	3.26%
MARKETING			
Advertising/Sales	**1.17%**	**0.89%**	0.88%
STOCK MANAGEMENT			
Stock Turn – Dispensary	**17.16**	**18.90**	N/A
Stock Turn – Retail	**2.97**	**2.39**	N/A
Stock Turn – Total	**7.15**	**7.36**	6.21
PRODUCTIVITY			
Floor Space			
Gross Profit Return per Square Meter	**$4,127**	**$3,725**	$3,326
Stock			
Gross Profit Return on Inventory Investment (GMROII)	**$3.29**	**$3.52**	$3.03

When moving towards a patient care practice, it will become very helpful to establish KPIs that are useful in measuring the performance and productivity of a patient care practice. This will allow you to evaluate how your patient care practice compares to other core business categories and its contribution to total net worth of the business.

In a community practice setting, comparing total sales per square foot of space devoted to patient services with prescription or other product sales may not be a very useful comparison. This is because the dollar volume of prescription and product sales may be significantly higher than dollar sales of patient services. Instead, you may want to look at the gross profit per square meter or net profit per square meter for a truer indicator of the activity's worth. If the actual space used is not an issue, then payroll costs will typically represent your greatest single operating expense after drug purchases. In this case, you may want to calculate the net profit generated per dollar invested in staff wages for patient care versus prescription sales.

Whatever benchmarks you eventually use to track the financial performance and success of your patient care services, you will need to either establish or interpret accounting data. However, you may still feel rather overwhelmed by the thought of tackling this complex process. Don't be. Remember the most critical part is for you to grasp the concepts and logic so you can extract the information that you need to manage your area.

This chapter was not intended to prepare you for a career in accounting. Rather, the intent was to give you a better understanding of the key concepts critical to financial management of patient services. If necessary, seek advice from financial advisors and accountants. With the knowledge you have gained from this chapter, you should be able to brief them properly and then understand and implement their advice.

References

1. Johnson JA, Bootman JL. Drug-related morbidity and mortality: a cost-of illness model. *Arch Intern Med*. 1995;155(18):1949-56.

Chapter 9
MANAGING PATIENT OUTCOME DATA
Kathleen A. Johnson & Karen B. Farris

Having access to patient information and gathering data that demonstrate positive patient outcomes is probably more important for pharmacists now, as they expand their role in health care, than it's ever been. Inappropriate drug use is expensive and harmful to patients, as several recent reports point out.[1-3] It's increasingly evident that the public, policy makers, and the medical community are ready for pharmacists to take a more proactive role in assuring health care quality and maximizing outcomes of medication use.

Although the ultimate benefit of gathering and managing patient data is continuity of care, another key reason why pharmacists should take on these responsibilities is because good data make it possible to evaluate the impact of pharmacist care and services on patient outcomes. Several research efforts demonstrate the value of pharmacist services, especially in institutional settings, but relatively few have been conducted in community pharmacies using adequate scientific rigor.[4-8] Consequently, it remains important to collect data that demonstrate the benefits of pharmacists' services, particularly in community settings and across the continuum of care.

Lately the focus on quality of care in managed care programs has been increasing. The National Committee for Quality Assurance (NCQA) requires reports from managed care health plans and physicians on quality of care measures such as structure, process, and outcome of care.[9] Employers and health plans use these measures to determine the benefits of medical care. Pharmacists are in a prime position to help providers and health plans achieve quality of care goals. Several NCQA quality measures are related to appropriate drug use and can be supported and improved by pharmacists.

Most patients have choices when it comes to health care plans and providers, including community pharmacies and hospitals. Pharmacists seeking managed care contracts and provider referrals must be able to supply information about the merits of their services through actual data—including the number of patients served, types of interventions made, and benefits and outcomes achieved. Patient data can support business marketing activities, as well.

Providers, patients, and health plans want to achieve the best outcomes possible from health care services while maintaining economic efficiency. Often, pharmaceuticals can be substituted for more expensive procedures and surgery. Services provided by pharmacists may be less expensive or more cost-effective than services provided in other health care settings. Pharmacists can use patient data to demonstrate the economic benefit of care, goods, and services provided in pharmacies. These data may also justify expanding services or making capital expenditures for larger facilities, remodeling, automation, equipment, or supplies.

As suggested earlier, collecting patient data and recording findings, interventions, problem assessments, and plans for resolution assure continuity of care, especially when multiple pharmacists are involved. These data also help pharmacists assure that therapy goals are achieved and allow them to provide timely and appropriate patient follow-up.

As a manager, patient outcome data are helpful to you in several ways. They allow you to make optimal use of personnel and facilities and, should consolidation or downsizing of operations be looming, they help you determine the possible impact. You may be able to use patient outcome data to gauge whether staff are following appropriate policies and procedures. Data can also be an invaluable tool when you are developing new operational systems or seeking effective methods to deliver patient care.

There are many reasons to keep good records of patient care data, including the most fundamental one—complying with legal and regulatory standards. Should a legal issue or malpractice suit arise, having an organized method in place for maintaining data will be a huge asset. Furthermore, health care payers require that records of services provided be available for audits. And capitated pharmaceutical care contracts may use patient management data to decide on future contracts or payment levels.

Types of Data

The types of patient care data you should maintain fall into seven broad categories:

1. Drug experience.
2. Clinical indicators of health status and disease control.
3. Humanistic.
4. Patient satisfaction.
5. Economic.
6. Service.
7. Procedural compliance.

Demonstrating interventions that have a positive impact on drug use and collecting relevant data are key ways to show the effectiveness of pharmacist services for improving outcomes. But the burden of data gathering—which may fall on not only the pharmacist but the patient and others—must be considered carefully. How much data do you need to generate needed reports and manage outcomes? There is no reason to collect data that are not going to be used.

Drug Experience Data

Pharmacists are probably most familiar with collecting drug-related data. The box to the right lists the seven types of drug therapy problems that Charles Hepler and Linda Strand have urged pharmacists to watch for and correct.[10] You must document the number and nature of drug therapy problems identified, the steps taken to resolve them, and the outcome.

Categories of Drug Therapy Problems

1. Unnecessary drug.
2. Lack of effectiveness (wrong drug).
3. Dosage too low.
4. Safety issues.
5. Dosage too high.
6. Compliance issues.
7. Untreated indication for a drug.

Adapted from Hepler CD, Strand LM. Opportunities and responsibilities in pharmaceutical care. *Am J Hosp Pharm.* 1990;47:533-43.

Collecting data on prescribing patterns is also useful. Data on the use of antibiotics, for example, can provide information about patterns of disease or prescriber treatment patterns for various indications or types of patients. Prescribing patterns may be of interest to pharmaceutical companies or health plans, as well.

Information regarding formulary compliance may also be useful. Formularies, whether open or closed, are often used to control the prescribing of high-cost treatment and to encourage the use of treatments that payers deem "preferred." To comply with the formulary, you must select treatments from a list of available agents in a drug class. This not only helps managed care plans and third-party payers control health care costs but may yield them better prices for medications or higher rebates from drug companies if certain measures of performance are achieved. Adhering to the formulary also lowers prescription prices for patients because their health plan covers the drugs they are prescribed.

Clinical Indicators of Health Status and Disease Control

Ongoing collection of patient data can demonstrate both positive and negative changes in health status and disease management over time, as well as any other changes resulting from pharmacist interventions. Tracking patients' symptoms helps you monitor disease control and motivate patients to improve their compliance with lifestyle and drug therapy. Laboratory studies, of course, are important clinical indicators of disease control, but patient complaints and symptoms can be key indicators, as well.

For hypertension, a clinical indicator of disease control would be blood pressure readings consistently at goal or within normal limits; patient symptoms may be vague or nonexistent no matter how poorly their hypertension is being managed. For asthma, peak expiratory flow readings that are at least 80% of the patient's best reading would be an important indicator of control but so would significant reductions in the severity and frequency of wheezing, cough, and breathing difficulty at different points in time. Whether laboratory measures or patient symptoms are useful indicators of health status and disease control depends on the condition. The same is true of their usefulness for monitoring patient progress over time. During periods of pharmacist intervention and management, you should record the appropriate data for each patient periodically and consistently to assess patient outcomes.

Humanistic Data

Despite clinicians' reliance on objective laboratory data or subjective patient complaints, signs, and symptoms, what matters most to patients are outcomes that affect their perception of general health and their ability to function in daily activities. These types of outcomes are growing in use as measures of the impact of health programs or medical care. The body of research on the usefulness and measurement of health-related quality of life outcomes is growing steadily.

Another type of outcome important to employers and patients is productivity and missed days from work, school, or normal activities. Changes in patient health behaviors (lifestyle and medication use) are also useful indicators of pharmacists' impact. Several approaches can be used to collect and evaluate humanistic data.

Health-Related Quality of Life

Quality of life may be measured as either general or disease-specific, both of which are assessed through either a verbal survey or written questionnaire. A common approach—but probably the least useful—is to ask a single question about how the patient perceives his or her overall quality of life.[11] This approach uses a scale, like a thermometer, to identify a level of health-related quality of life at the time of survey. It can be useful, but is so general that you risk capturing concepts other than health-related quality of life, such as a side effect from treatment, a bad day, or simply frustration with some aspect of health care or treatment.

John Ware and colleagues developed the Short-Form 36 (SF-36) and the scaled-down 12 item SF-12 questionnaires to measure quality of life.[12] Validated as general health-related quality of life measures, they divide quality of life into two primary domains: physical function and mental function. The advantage of using a general health-related quality of life instrument is that people with various conditions or diseases can be compared with each other over time.

Disease-Specific Quality of Life

Disease-specific quality of life measures are relevant to a particular disease or condition. The most useful tool would measure both patient- and disease-specific health status, be sensitive to improvement or worsening of the disease, and capture both negative and positive effects of treatment. Ideally, disease-specific measures of quality of life should be correlated with clinical measures of disease severity, but they are still often susceptible to how the patient perceives the effect of treatment on his or her personal health status and role functioning.

Several disease-specific survey instruments have been validated to capture improvements and worsening of a variety of chronic diseases, including asthma, hypertension, diabetes, and gastrointestinal disease.[13] A disadvantage of disease-specific measures of quality of life is that only people with the same medical condition can be compared with each other. To overcome this problem, researchers will often combine a disease-specific instrument with a general health-related quality of life survey.

Pharmacists providing patient services are in an ideal situation to periodically assess changes in general or disease-specific quality of life. To properly use quality of life surveys and collect these data, it's best to work in consultation with someone familiar with the various surveys available, domains of interest, and proper scoring. A good place to find such assistance is your local college of pharmacy, where a knowledgeable researcher may be willing to help you gather data—especially if the data relate to one of the researcher's projects or areas of interest. Many quality of life instruments are copyrighted. You may need permission to use them, which can make their cost prohibitive for routine use.

Missed Days and Productivity

Employers are increasingly concerned with absenteeism and reduced productivity as measures of the quality and effectiveness of health care programs. Parents and students worry about missed days at school because of the risk of academic failure. You can capture data about lost work days, reduced productivity, and school absenteeism as a measure of the benefits of health care and pharmacists' services. These data can easily be gathered during pharmacy visits or inpatient stays, or when medications are dispensed.

Productivity and missed days from work or school are important to some segments of the population, but everyone wants to participate in normal daily activities, carry out role functions, and maintain leisure pursuits. Don't overlook these areas when measuring the results of improved disease control and pharmacist services. Often they are assessed by simple questions about the person's role functioning, productivity, and enjoyment of usual leisure activities.[11]

Health Behaviors

Ultimately, patient health behaviors influence how patients seek health care, participate in preventive care options, and follow the advice of health care professionals to achieve optimal outcomes. The health belief model is a useful framework for predicting the behavior of consumers based on various external and internal influences.[14] You should be familiar with this model to understand and influence health behaviors—those things people do to improve or maintain their health. Health behaviors are the actions of individuals, groups, and organizations and the things that cause, are related to, or result from those actions.[15] Once you identify behaviors in need of change, an important part of managing patient outcome data is proving that the behavior has been changed.

The most critical health behavior related to medication use is taking the medication as instructed—known as "adherence" or "compliance." Improper use of medication has been identified as a major public health problem, which pharmacists can play a primary role in addressing. Donald Morisky and colleagues[16] have developed and validated a four-item patient questionnaire to measure compliance based on self-reported patient responses. Other measures of compliance include counting pills left in containers, asking patients how they take their medication and comparing it to the directions for use, and checking for on-time refills.

The medication–possession ratio (number of doses available based on actual refills, divided by the number of doses that should be available based on directions for use) gives the percentage of time that patients have appropriate amounts of medications available for use. The ratio score ranges from 0 to 1. A score of 1 means that 100% of the time, the number of doses refilled corresponds exactly to the number of doses that should have been refilled.[17]

A practical aspect of compliance that pharmacists should take into account is a person's ability to manage his or her medications. Medication management involves having and applying the psychomotor and cognitive skills to take medications as directed.[18] Visual acuity, cognitive ability, fine motor skills, memory, and the ability to understand and remember instructions contribute to the capacity to manage medication regimens effectively and without error.[19-22] Age-related changes in physical functioning, sensory acuity, and cognition that are prevalent in older people can make medication management difficult for this population, especially when regimens are complex.[23,24] You should consider medication management ability as one specific aspect of medication compliance and collect data to indicate deficiencies and improvement in this area.

You can also help patients adopt health behaviors that are generally recommended as beneficial and measure changes in these health behaviors over time. Among these types of behaviors are:

+ Lifestyle, such as exercise and diet.
+ Self-monitoring of blood glucose and other measures.
+ Self care, such as periodically checking feet to identify sores and ulcerations.
+ Learning about the disease or treatment to acquire knowledge of drug therapy side effects or proper use of medications.

Recommended behaviors should be individualized for the patient's condition. During work-ups and consultations, evaluate and document patients' health behaviors to identify patient education opportunities and assess the impact of your interventions over time.

Patient Satisfaction

Health plans and employers are increasingly interested in assessing patient satisfaction with medical care, including pharmacist services. The two types of pharmacy services for which satisfaction can be measured are:

+ Dispensing and counseling services.
+ Cognitive services.

Traditionally, patient satisfaction surveys have focused on dispensing[25,26] and have been administered in writing at the time services are obtained or shortly thereafter. John Ware and colleagues have developed and validated a satisfaction instrument for medical care[27] from which components have been adapted to measure patient satisfaction with consulting and other pharmacist services.[28] Recently, Lon Larson and colleagues developed an instrument to assess satisfaction with pharmaceutical care services.[29]

Economic Data

Economic data are useful not only for evaluating medication costs, health service utilization, and operational costs, but also for assessing patient outcomes. When evaluating economic data, keep in mind the perspective of the organization or entity for whom "value" is to be demonstrated. For example, you need to consider the hospital's perspective when demonstrating pharmacists' value to a hospital. The hospital administration is likely to be most interested in the costs associated with providing care in the hospital and less interested in physician office visits or costs to the patient or insurance company, but the latter three areas would be very important when evaluating the impact of services provided in a community pharmacy.

The economic arrangements concerning payment for products or services also influence the outcomes that interest health care providers and payers. For example,

CASE EXAMPLE: Asthma Care Service

Pharmacy ABC has a new asthma care service. This service is expected to improve patient use and compliance with inhaler medications for asthma control, reduce unnecessary use of rescue inhalers, increase patient self-monitoring with peak-flow meters, and develop asthma medication action plans in conjunction with patients' physicians. The action plan tells patients what to do when asthma symptoms worsen or when they are exposed to an asthma trigger. The service is based on guidelines from the National Institutes of Health for optimal asthma control. Following these guidelines has been demonstrated to improve long-term patient outcomes, reduce unnecessary emergency room visits and hospitalizations, and improve the quality of care. This service is paid for by the People's Managed Care Company from funds designated for medical care services. Consider the perspective or financial incentives of each of the following:

The medical specialist (pulmonologist) paid on a fee-for-service basis.
The hospital contracted to provide services to People's Managed Care Company enrollees, which is economically at risk if hospitalization is overused.
The medical group, which is capitated for patient care and is at risk if use of the emergency room, hospitalization, or drugs is too high.

a capitated medical group that receives payments as a per-person monthly fee regardless of the services provided typically places each provider at financial risk for improper or excessive use of pharmaceuticals. Such an arrangement can be devastating if the medical group is responsible for the cost of outpatient drug use beyond a predetermined amount. Providers in capitated contracts will definitely hold a different view of economic data than a medical group that is primarily paid on a fee-for-service or discounted fee-for-service basis with no risk for hospital or pharmaceutical expenses. To illustrate this point, let's examine the case above.

Based on the way the People's Managed Care Company pays each of the groups in the example, how would they view the new asthma care service? The medical specialist may view it as competition, whereas the hospital would welcome services that avoid excessive utilization. The medical group would be in favor of it as well, as long as the physicians feel comfortable with the pharmacists' qualifications and confident that the pharmacists will maintain proper communication about their patients.

All health care providers and organizations want improved patient outcomes and a high quality of care, but you should also consider the financial picture when using data to justify new services or programs or when seeking "buy-in" from collaborators.

Medication Costs

A common type of economic data evaluated in conjunction with pharmacist services is the cost of medications and pharmaceutical-related products, including prescription and nonprescription drugs, durable medical equipment, and patient supplies such as bandages and glucose meter strips. These data would be used when the payer or provider is concerned with the added financial expense of such items or when it's important to determine a program's impact on compliance with prescribed drug therapy or other treatment regimens.

There is one caveat in the use of "medication cost" data. Frequently, managed care health plans have special or contract prices that are confidential or they receive rebates that are not disclosed and therefore cannot be factored into the actual purchase price of prescription drugs. Therefore, it is common to use the average wholesale price (AWP) as an estimate of product cost. Cost information can be estimated from claims data, especially since most prescription payment programs base pharmacy payment in part on AWP minus a percentage plus a fee. But if you have access to actual cost data you are in a better position to measure true economic impact related to medication costs.

Health Service Utilization

Health service utilization data most often relate to frequency of visits to emergency rooms, urgent care centers, and physician offices as well as numbers of hospitalizations and lengths of hospital stays. Sometimes, depending on the purpose of the service and the perspective you're evaluating, data on laboratory costs, intermediate- and long-term care admissions, dental office visits, hospice care, physical therapy, and use of other services are also relevant.

It can be difficult to collect these data unless you have access to claims data files. Patients tend to have poor recall about their use of health services except for unusual or major events such as a hospitalization or emergency room visit. Even a hospitalization can be forgotten and dates of hospital admission and discharge can be remembered incorrectly.

Claims data can pose problems, too. For example, data based on payment for services provided can be inaccurate if each patient visit is not recorded properly. In capitated medical groups, where claims are not submitted for services provided (and thus the medical plan does not receive information about each visit or procedure), data about patient encounters can also be inaccurate or missing. The person collecting data about health services must be familiar with inherent irregularities, including potential missing data.

When assigning costs for health care utilization, you should use the "paid" claim amount for a service rather than the amount charged (submitted on the bill). Even though the provider submits a bill for a service, the amount paid more closely reflects the payer's value of that service and thus it is the appropriate cost data for most purposes.

If encounter data rather than actual paid claims are available, you can use literature-based references to assign costs, such as the average charge for a day in the hospital or the usual capitated payment for a specific diagnosis. Because patient confidentiality must be maintained, it is difficult to obtain claims data linked directly to patients.

Operational Costs

The easiest economic data to obtain are those collected routinely by your own operational systems, including prescriptions filled per day, labor costs, type of personnel employed, nonprescription sales data, and lease or space costs. You can access these data without any special permission or constraints and, unlike claims data, they are probably in a familiar format. A key use of such data is to analyze the costs of providing a new service. For more information on operational costs, see Chapter 8.

Service Data

Service data relate to frequency, quality, and procedural compliance for such services as providing drug information consults to physicians, consulting with patients, resolving drug therapy problems, making nonprescription product recommendations, handling patient triage and referral, offering disease management services, and completing laboratory tests.

Frequency

Data in this category have to do with the frequency of patient contact, such as asthma care visits or patient counseling encounters. It's easy to obtain the first kind of data from the patient's chart or the appointment record, but the second kind is less likely to be recorded or documented, even though patient counseling may be provided more routinely than asthma care.

To collect data on both the number of sessions and the length of each session, you must put special procedures in place. Possible collection methods, depending on how accurate you must be, include direct observation, completing a data form for each session, or videotaping the session. You also need to consider the cost of each method. Pilot-test your service encounter forms before you put them into regular use to be sure that they can be completed accurately and that they cover the proper categories of information. When necessary, be sure that staff members who will collect these data receive training in completing the forms accurately. Later, this chapter will discuss data collection methods more fully.

Quality

The quality of health care services is typically described in terms of structural measures, process measures, and outcome measures.[9, 30-32] Using the asthma care service as an example, quality could be measured structurally by the types of equipment available and the credentials of the pharmacist or personnel providing the service. Process measures include how the actual care is provided and the appropriateness of patient education techniques. Outcome measures gauge the patient's improvement by looking at such things as reduced emergency room visits, lessened symptoms, or increased compliance. Obviously, each of these quality measures provides a different level of data.

Structural measures are the easiest to obtain but the least likely to be associated with true health care quality. Certainly, the training of personnel and availability of equipment are important for quality care, but the process by which care is actually provided is even more important and more highly correlated with actual quality. Patient outcomes, although more difficult and costly to measure than structure and process, provide the ultimate demonstration of high-quality care. Early programs for quality assurance and accreditation focused more on structural measures, but emphasis has now shifted to process and outcome measures.

Procedural Compliance

Independent accreditation and evaluation organizations exist to ensure that the providers of health care services—both personnel and entities such as hospitals, health plans, and medical groups—are properly qualified. The entities interested in assuring that care givers follow appropriate procedures are payers, employers, consumers, and the federal government. The Joint Commission on Accreditation of Healthcare Organizations (JCAHO) and the National Committee for Quality Assurance (NCQA) are most relevant to hospitals or ambulatory care and community pharmacies, respectively.

Hospital pharmacists have long been familiar with the JCAHO process to ensure that institutional services are of sufficient quality. Community pharmacies offering home infusion services have also been required to meet JCAHO standards for accreditation.

NCQA was designed to give employer groups feedback about the quality of care provided through managed care health plans. The Health Evaluation Data Information Set (HEDIS) is a set of standards put forth by NCQA that are often used by managed care plans to evaluate the care that medical groups provide to plan members. Because many of the HEDIS measures lend themselves to pharmacist intervention, an opportunity exists for pharmacists to help health plans and medical groups achieve NCQA/HEDIS quality goals if they are given the proper payment incentives. There is an increasing trend to develop standards, to measure against them the care provided, and to provide this information to consumers and payers so they can make informed choices.[9,33] In response to the Institute of Medicine report on errors in medicine,[3] some states are mandating quality assurance programs in pharmacies so as to reduce medication errors.[34]

The Food and Drug Administration requirement that pharmaceutical companies report adverse drug events (ADEs) is another example of procedural compliance relevant to pharmacy. To improve patient safety, pharmaceutical manufacturers must conduct phase IV postmarketing surveillance studies that monitor and evaluate ADEs. Hospital pharmacists have participated in the reporting process as part of JCAHO accreditation, and more recently community pharmacists have started reporting ADEs and product-specific problems. Data collected by pharmacists on the frequency and type of ADEs have tremendous value for selecting drugs and for gauging how effectively pharmacist services influence appropriate therapy.

Data Collection Techniques

This section gives you an overview of useful statistical tools. Although you may be working with a researcher who is responsible for the actual "number crunching," it's helpful to understand the terminology and techniques. The most important thing to remember is that data you collect should never be accepted at face value; it needs to be interpreted using appropriate statistical techniques.

Before collecting data it's important to consider why you want the data in the first place. For example, if you plan to evaluate the impact of your care on patient outcomes, you may be able to use clinical information in your pharmacy care records that was gathered to monitor a specific drug-related issue or disease parameter. You may have records on the number of elevated blood sugars or on pain ratings according to a pain scale, for instance. Your data collection then becomes a simple process of abstracting specific information from your pharmacy care records. However, if you want to know whether the person's quality of life improved, you probably did not collect the pertinent data during routine patient care. You would have to devise a mechanism for collecting that type of data. Creating your own survey is not a good idea unless you have specific expertise in this area; you may find yourself measuring something other than what you think you're measuring. The best route is to use a published survey that has been appropriately validated, and ask your patients to complete it at a specific time and place.

Variables and Level of Measurement

Before discussing data collection further, it may be helpful to review some definitions. A variable is a logical grouping of attributes. Attributes are characteristics of persons or things.[35] For example, sex is a logical grouping of the attributes "male" and "female." A code is the number assigned to the attributes. For the variable "sex," 1 could be assigned to the attribute "female" and 2 could be assigned to the attribute "male."

You might have blood glucose control as the variable in question, and the attribute would be the number of times in a week that fasting readings exceed the normal range. With this information, you could then define someone's diabetes as controlled or uncontrolled.

There are different levels of measurement that are important to consider when selecting specific variables to evaluate.[35] A *nominal* variable has attributes that are simply categories with no order, such as "male" and "female." The categories of an *ordinal* variable have order, but the difference between the categories may not be the same, such as "always," "sometimes," and "never." An *interval* variable has categories of attributes with quantifiable differences, such as 10%, 20%, 30%, and so on.

Using blood glucose monitoring as an example, Table 9-1 illustrates these concepts. A patient's frequency of blood glucose monitoring can be an ordinal variable if you ask him or her to respond using "never," "sometimes," "frequently," or "all the time." It is easy to see that "frequently" is more than "sometimes," but it is not clear if the difference between "all the time" and "frequently" is equivalent to the difference between "sometimes" and "never."

You can also ask patients to tell you the number of times they test their blood sugar each day, and then use that information to calculate the number of times per week. If they test their blood sugar four times per day, then that is two times more than if they test it twice a day. This would be an interval variable, because there is a quantifiable difference between the categories of 0, 1, 2, 3, and so on.

Yet another type of measurement, *ratio*, is similar to interval except that it has a true zero. Interval and ratio data are generally more desirable because they can be used in more powerful statistical techniques. Furthermore, an interval variable can always be converted into an ordinal or nominal variable, but not vice versa. For example, if you identify the actual number of times patients check their blood glucose, you could define them as "conscientious" if it's 21 times per week, "needs encouragement" if it's 20 to 14 times per week, and "needs improvement" if it's fewer than 14 times per week. You could then assign each person to one of these three categories and develop communications and programs targeted specifically to each category. After delivering a program you could determine if you were able to move people from the "needs improvement" category to the "conscientious" category.

Although level of measurement probably sounds like technical research jargon with no relevance to you, it's something you must consider during data collection. It is imperative that you use the correct level of measurement with the correct statistical procedure when you analyze your data. If you are unclear about the type of data to collect, it is generally safe to collect interval level data, which can be converted into nominal or ordinal variables.

Table 9-1. Examples of Level of Measurement

	Variable Name	Data to Collect	Variable Definition	Code in the Data Set
Nominal	Blood glucose control	Number of times in a week FBG is not within normal range; number of FBGs in the week	Percent of FBGs within normal range. Considered controlled if the percent is 90% or greater.	1= Yes; 90% or greater 0 = No; less than 90%
Ordinal	Blood glucose control	Number of times in a week FBG is not within normal range; number of FBGs in the week	Levels of control = Never = 0-33% Sometimes = 34-65% Frequently = 66-89% All the time = 90% or greater	1 = Never 2 = Sometimes 3 = Frequently 4 = All the time
Interval	Blood glucose control	Number of times in a week FBG is not within normal range; number of FBGs in the week	Percent of FBGs within normal range	Percent of FBGs within normal range

FBG = fasting blood glucose

Sources of Data

Generally, there are four primary sources of data you should consider in answering specific questions. Each of these sources, listed below, has strengths and weaknesses regarding cost and ease of collection, which are summarized in Table 9-2.

+ Pharmacy records.
+ Patients or their representatives.
+ Other providers.
+ Secondary data, such as prescription orders or insurance claims.

Table 9-2. Characteristics of Data Sources

Data Source	Ease	Cost
Pharmacy records	Very easy	Inexpensive
Patients or their representatives	Doable	Expensive
Other providers	Doable, but more difficult	Expensive
Secondary data	Can be difficult; dependent on others	Can be expensive, especially if not in your contract

Pharmacy Records

Pharmacy records contain data that you have gathered directly or that were given to you in the normal course of pharmacy practice. These records may consist of patient care information, prescriptions, financial data, or human resource data. In terms of patient-centered pharmacy management, documenting patient care can be a valuable source of data for examining who uses services, the effectiveness of services and care, and even reimbursement amounts.

An important aspect of patient care records is that they describe the people in your analyses. In other words, not only do you collect variables that tell you if your program is effective, but you also collect demographic variables that describe the people in the program. It will not be sufficient to say that people in your program, for example, use on average four prescription medications. You will also want to know other information such as age, gender, and concurrent diagnoses. When assessing the effectiveness of services, you must document goals for patients and then reassess them to determine the extent to which goals have been met. These goals and whether they have been met can then be summarized across a group of patients. Staffing records may also be useful to consider when examining trends in dispensing errors, for example.

A key piece of advice: before you collect more data, think about whether you can answer your questions with data you already have in your pharmacy. Using data that are already collected has some disadvantages, but it can also have advantages, such as saving time and money.

Patients

Patients or their representatives provide you with information during your care for them, but that is not the type of information we're referring to here. Using patients as a source of data means collecting additional information that would not be collected in normal pharmacy practice. A patient satisfaction survey is a good example. You probably don't typically ask patients whether they expect you to phone them 5 days after they get a new prescription filled. But if you ask this question in an anonymous survey distributed with all new prescriptions during a 2-week period, you may learn something important that you can do for patients.

In addition to surveys distributed at the pharmacy, patients can be interviewed in person or by telephone. In such interviews, the interviewer usually knows the name of the interviewee, which, depending on the issue, may be a conflict of interest. If you called your patients directly and asked if they are happy with the amount of patient counseling they receive and the approaches used, they would have a hard time being honest. And their responses could affect the way they are treated in the future. (See ethical issues on page 200 in this chapter.)

Other Providers

Other providers can be an important source of data, especially when you are seeking information to help you determine the impact of your services. Or you may be interested in the opinion of other providers about your patient-centered services. In either case, a survey or focus group may give you good insights.

Secondary Data

Secondary data is a general term referring to data used for research that was collected for another purpose. A classic example is prescription claims. These records are filed and maintained for both legal and reimbursement reasons, but you could also use them to determine how many patients on cholesterol-lowering medications in the past 6 months were either late in getting their refill or did not get their refill at all. In other words, prescription claims can be used to identify people who might benefit from an educational, compliance, reminder, or support program.

Data Collection Timeframe

The timeframe for data collection depends on the information you are seeking. You may be trying to answer some question in the past, such as "What was the apparent impact of the radio advertising that we ran last Christmas?" Or you may want to provide a service and then evaluate it as you go along, or perhaps at 3 months after you provided it. Answering a question with data collected in the past is generally known as a *retrospective* study. Collecting data as one implements a program is often referred to as a *concurrent* or *prospective* study. Each data collection method has advantages and disadvantages.

Retrospective Data Collection

The primary strength of retrospective data is that it is already collected, which generally makes it less expensive to access. Costs associated with accessing retrospective data, however, vary depending on the source. When using your own pharmacy records, the costs may be limited to paying someone to go through the records and abstract what is needed. If, however, you are asking your computer vendor or information systems division to provide retrospective data about the frequency of ACE inhibitor refills, you will probably have to pay for computer and programming time. Using retrospective data to which you do not have direct access usually costs money because the data's owner incurs expenses in pulling together the specific data you want.

Prospective Data Collection

Collecting data on an ongoing basis to be analyzed sometime in the future is prospective data collection. Suppose you want to implement a program to track dispensing errors made in the pharmacy. You plan how to do it and invest in the appropriate training for your staff.

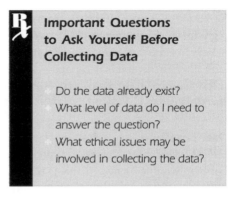

Important Questions to Ask Yourself Before Collecting Data

Do the data already exist?
What level of data do I need to answer the question?
What ethical issues may be involved in collecting the data?

You may decide to have technicians document the prescription number, patient name, drug name, type of error, date, time of error, time of error recognition, mode of error recognition, pharmacist making the error, and the pharmacist identifying the error. These records can be kept in a computer database or a paper binder so that twice a year you can examine monthly trends.

Ongoing data collection is valuable to managers because it lets you assess the impact of your programs and services, ascertain whether goals and objectives are being met, and answer other questions that may arise in the future.

Cross-Sectional and Time Series

A cross-sectional approach to data collection means that you gather data for one point in time. For example, if you are surveying customers about their satisfaction with your pharmacy services, you might conduct the survey in September, although you are asking about their satisfaction over the previous 3 months. Alternatively, you could ask them every 6 months to report how satisfied they are. In the latter approach, known as a time series, you collect data at specified points in time and examine the trends in the numbers. An example of time-series data that may be pertinent to pharmacists providing care to older people is cognitive or functional status scores. You might obtain such information quarterly from nurses or occupational therapists.

Do the Data Exist?

If the data you want already exist, either in your pharmacy or in a secondary data set such as insurance records, determine the cost of accessing these data before you start collecting new data. It is generally less expensive, either in direct costs or time, to use data that have already been collected. You have to consider, however, whether the existing data are in a format that is compatible with your needs. If you are interested in medication dispensing errors and your documentation system fails to record the time and circumstances of error identification, it may not be feasible for you to examine trends in how errors are detected. You may be limited to identifying when the error actually occurred, but not when it was identified—which may or may not be the same time. Thus, just because data on dispensing medication errors is kept doesn't mean it is compatible with your needs. In such cases, you should consider changing the type of data collected or collecting your own data to meet your specific needs.

Data Level

The level of data you need is determined by what you want to know or the question you want to answer. There is no right or wrong here. If you are happy knowing the range of times that a person monitors blood glucose, such as 1–5 or 10–15 times per week, then that level of measurement (ordinal data) is fine. From a research perspective, interval data are the most desirable, but collecting interval data can be a burden and may not be necessary if, for example, you are looking at quality of care in your pharmacy. But if you are going to use the data to demonstrate outcomes, negotiate payment contracts, or support marketing initiatives, then most likely you will need to collect interval data.

Ethical Issues

Among the ethical issues you must consider when collecting data[35,36]:

+ **Confidentiality and privacy**. Confidentiality means that you know the identities of the people giving you information, but you agree not to share them with others. You can share the information as long as individuals cannot be identified. In contrast, privacy means that you will keep secret any sensitive, personal information that your patients give you. If data are anonymous you do not know who provided them, although you may know information that characterizes them. For example, you may know that a 45-year-old female with osteoarthritis answered the survey, but you do not know the name of the woman who completed it.
+ **Respect for people**. Respecting others implies that people have an opportunity to determine the data they want to provide. Even though patient care data may be accessible to you, collecting additional data that do not relate directly to care requires that patients give their approval.
+ **Beneficence**. This means that the benefits to the patient of participating in a given program or project outweigh the risks.

It is incumbent on you to keep any data you collect from patients or providers private and confidential. You know that you shouldn't tell one neighbor the medications that another neighbor is taking, and the same principle applies to data you collect. If patients agree for you to share data with their physicians, for example, then you have fulfilled your obligation of privacy and confidentiality by seeking this explicit exception.

It is also your responsibility to know who can view data that you have collected and to make sure that those people understand the issues regarding privacy and confidentiality. For example, will your secretary or staff pharmacists have access to the data you collect regarding patient satisfaction?

Data should be securely stored by way of locked cabinets, computer passwords, or other safe means. If you are analyzing data to identify trends or detect differences according to such characteristics as age or sex, it is advisable to omit patients' names in that data set. You can assign each patient a study identification number and keep a list of patient names with their corresponding numbers in a separate, locked place. Then, even if people see your data, they can't tell who it specifically represents.

As for respect, if you are collecting information not needed for patient care, patients have the right to withhold it. In fact, some patients may refuse even to provide care information you want, and that is their right. Patients may also choose to answer some questions and not others. Their participation in projects must be voluntary.

Beneficence suggests that people participating in your project or receiving your interventions are the ones likely to benefit. The benefits outweigh the risks. Projects in community pharmacies are not likely to cause significant immediate risks, but it may be difficult to assess the long-term risks. If the project involves clinical trials or invasive procedures, then some risks do exist and patients must be fully informed.

If you are involved in a research project associated with a university, always ensure that ethical approval for the study has been obtained. Projects involving human subjects must be approved by the institutional review board, which examines proposed research to ensure the benefits outweigh the risks, before they can proceed. Depending on the scope of the project, informed consent may be required from your research subjects. Form 9-1 is an example of an informed consent form for a community pharmacy-based project. The appendix at the end of this chapter gives an example of a study information sheet.

There are several principles you should consider as you begin data collection, most of which need little explanation. It is better to collect a few variables completely and accurately than to collect many variables but with incomplete data. Do not try to answer in one study or analysis every research question you have. Be specific and limit your research question, thereby limiting your variables and analyses. All data need to be collected for all participants. When data are input into a spreadsheet, check carefully for accuracy. The box on page 203 lists key principles related to data collection.

Form 9-1. Patient Group A, Informed Consent

**Title: Health care outcomes of senior Albertans
after the provision of pharmaceutical care**

Principal Investigator:
Roger Research, PharmD, Assistant Professor
Phone: 555-123-4567
Co-investigators:
Sally Study, MD, Assistant Professor
Phone: 555-234-5678
Nick Numbercruncher, PhD, Assistant Professor
Phone: 555-345-6789

	Yes	No
Do you understand that you have been asked to be in a research study?	☐	☐
Have you read and received a copy of the attached Information Sheet?	☐	☐
Do you understand the benefits and risks of taking part in this research study?	☐	☐
Have you had an opportunity to ask questions and discuss this study?	☐	☐
Do you understand that you are free to withdraw from the study at any time, without having to give a reason and without affecting your future medical or pharmacy care?	☐	☐
Has the issue of confidentiality been explained to you?	☐	☐
Do you understand who will have access to your medical records?	☐	☐
Do you understand that your family doctor will know you are a part of this study?	☐	☐

Who explained this study to you?_____

I agree to take part in this study: ☐   ☐

Signature of research subject_____

Printed name_____ Date_____

Signature of witness_____

Signature of investigator or designee_____

Data Analysis and Reporting

Many research questions of interest to practicing pharmacists can be answered with relatively simple statistics you can calculate with a spreadsheet. There are generally two types of statistics: descriptive and inferential.[35] Descriptive statistics, used to summarize data, can answer many of the questions that practicing pharmacists have. Descriptive statistics typically tell about the distribution of a variable (frequency distribution) or its relationship with other variables (measures of association). The correct statistic to use and report, however, generally depends on the level of measurement: nominal, ordinal, ratio, or interval.

Descriptive Statistics

Frequency distribution, a term commonly used in descriptive statistics, is the number of cases having a specific attribute of a variable. Table 9-3 shows several variables that have been collected for 10 cases. The frequency distribution for the variable labeled "Sex" would be 5 for "1," which

 Principles in Data Collection

Collect a few variables well.

Be able to describe who provided the data using demographics and other descriptive information, such as age group and where the data came from (ages 45-49, members of health plan X, telephone interviews of patients with diabetes, etc.).

Collect the same data on all participants.

Pretest your data collection mechanisms.

Check for complete data collection. When possible, collect either interval or ratio data, which can be analyzed using more rigorous statistical tests than can be used on nominal or ordinal data.

Check a sample of data that has been input into your spreadsheet or database to be sure it is accurate.

Table 9-3. Sample Data Set*

Case No.	Sex	Age	Uses Insulin	Monitors per Day	Education Session	Times out of Range
1	1	65	1	3	0	7
2	2	85	0	1	1	10
3	1	72	1	4	1	6
4	2	81	1	2	1	6
5	1	68	1	2	1	4
6	2	77	0	4	0	0
7	2	67	1	3	1	15
8	1	73	1	3	1	3
9	1	80	1	2	0	12
10	2	79	0	3	1	9

* Taken from a larger data set.

Vocabulary Review: Statistics and Data Collection

Alpha: The level of significance required and determined in advance. An alpha of 0.05 means that you want to be 95% certain (1 minus alpha) that the difference you have measured is real (significant) and not due to random chance.

Attributes: Characteristics of people or things.

Chi-square test: Measures the significance of the difference between proportions. For example, you would use a chi-square test if you found that 56 out of 65 (56/65 is a proportion) patients were satisfied with one type of pharmacy service while 74 out of 88 (74/88) patients were satisfied with another type of service and you wanted to know if the difference between proportions was real or due to random chance.

Code: A number assigned to attributes.

Critical value: The threshold value of a statistical test that must be exceeded in order to reject the null hypothesis.

Cross-sectional study: A study in which data are collected for one point in time (such as patient satisfaction in the month of October).

Degrees of freedom: In inferential statistics, the amount of data used to calculate a statistic. For example, if you perform a measurement in 15 patients, you will have 14 degrees of freedom (sample size of 15 minus 1).

Descriptive statistics: A type of statistic used to summarize or describe data, such as mean, variance, standard deviation, etc.

Frequency distribution: The tally of the number of times each score occurs in a group of scores, such as twelve patients age 1–10 years, thirteen patients age 11–20 years, etc.

Inferential statistics: Uses tests based on probability theory to make generalizations from samples to the population from which the sample was taken. For example, you might determine that you are 95% certain that the average blood sugar measures of 88 mg/dl in Group One and 109 mg/dl in Group Two are actually different results and the difference is not due to random chance.

Interval variable: A measurement that describes variables in such a way that the distance between any two adjacent units of measurement (or "intervals") is the same, but in which there is no meaningful zero point.

Mean: The average value of a set of numbers.

Measure of dispersion: Describes how widely data are distributed. Common measures of dispersion are standard deviation and variance.

continued on page 205

Vocabulary Review: Statistics and Data Collection, continued

Measures of association: Describes the degree of relationship between two or more measurements (for example, the incidence of chronic disease is shown to be related to increased age).

Nominal variable: A level of measurement in which attributes are categories with no order, such as male and female.

Null hypothesis: An assumption in a statistical test that the difference between results is due to random chance and is not significant. Inferential statistics are used to reject (or fail to reject) the null hypothesis.

Ordinal variable: A level of measurement in which the categories of attributes have order but the difference between the categories may not be the same, such as always, sometimes, and never.

p value: Degree of certainty that two results are different. Differs from alpha in that it is determined from the data and is not determined in advance. For example, if $p = 0.05$, you can be 95% (1 minus p) certain that the results are truly different. If $p = 0.01$, then you are 99% certain.

Prospective or concurrent study: A study in which data are collected while the study is in progress.

Ratio variable: A level of measurement similar to interval variables, except it has a true zero. For example, theoretically a patient can have a blood pressure of zero (no blood pressure is present).

Retrospective study: A study that uses data collected in the past.

Standard deviation (SD): A measure of dispersion that describes how widely the results are distributed around the mean: for example, 68% of results fall +/– 1 SD, or 95% of results fall +/– 2 SD. SD is the square root of variance.

Time-series study: Gathers data multiple times (such as patient satisfaction every 6 months).

Variable: A logical grouping of attributes (such as age or gender).

Variance: A measure of dispersion equal to the square of the standard deviation. A small variance means that the data are clustered closely around the mean. Used less frequently than standard deviation because it is a less rigorous measurement.

stands for male, and 5 for "2," which stands for female. Therefore, the frequency distribution for sex can be expressed as 50% male and 50% female. For the variable "Uses Insulin" there are seven people coded "1" or yes and three people coded "0" or no. So the frequency of people who use insulin in our data set is 7 out of 10 or 70%. Nominal and ordinal data are reported using frequency distributions. As explained earlier, nominal data are grouped into categories such as male and female. Ordinal data are grouped into categories that have order but the difference between the categories may not be the same, such as "always," "sometimes," and "never." Thus the best way to report these data is to place them into frequency distributions that show how many data points are assigned to each category.

The mean of a variable is the arithmetic average of the values. Means can generally only be calculated for interval or ratio data. In Table 9-3 you can calculate the mean for the "Age" variable by adding all the ages together and dividing by the total number of cases, which is 10. The average age is $747 \div 10 = 74.7$.

When you calculate a mean, it is critical to also calculate a standard deviation (SD)—a measure of how widely the data are dispersed—so you know how much variation is in your data. SD is the square root of the variance, which is yet another measure of dispersion and is expressed as s^2. Variance is calculated by the following equation:

$$s^2 = \Sigma \, (x_1 - mean)^2 \div (n - 1)$$

Σ means "the sum of," x_1 is the particular value of some point of data, n is the total number of data points, and $n - 1$ is the number of degrees of freedom (df). Most scientific calculators can calculate the variance and SD of a set of data, so the equation is given here only for your information. The standard deviation is always reported with a mean and is represented as mean $+/-$ SD. If the standard deviation is large, the range between the highest and lowest data point is also going to be large. By definition, 68.26% of data fall $+/- 1$ SD from the mean and 95.44% of data fall $+/- 2$ SD from the mean.

The mean age of the subjects in Table 9-3 is 74.7 years and the SD is calculated as 6.7 years. Therefore, you can say that the mean age of the patients is 74.7 $+/- 6.7$ years. Because 68.26% of the subjects will have an age within 1 SD of the mean, 68.26% fall between the ages of 68.0 (mean $-$ SD) and 81.4 (mean $+$ SD).

Descriptive statistics can also be used to compare subgroups. For example, you could determine the average number of medications (the descriptive statistic) used by males and by females (subgroups). Referring to Table 9-3, you could calculate the average number of times blood glucose is monitored per day for those people who use insulin and for those who do not. First, add up the number of times people who use insulin monitor their blood glucose $(3 + 4 + 2 + 2 + 3 + 3 + 2 = 19)$. Then divide by the number of people who use insulin, which in this instance is 7. Thus the average is $19 \div 7 = 2.71$. Following the same steps, the average number of times per day that people not on insulin monitor their blood glucose is $(1 + 4 + 3) = 8 \div 3 = 2.67$. Therefore, patients who use insulin monitor their blood sugar on average 0.04 times more often per day than patients who do not use insulin $(2.71 - 2.67 = 0.04)$. Without using adequate statistical testing, we cannot tell if this difference is a real difference (what statisticians call a significant difference) or if the difference is simply due to random chance in the numbers. Inferential statistics tells you whether the difference is significant or random.

A good analogy would be to step on your bathroom scale and weigh yourself. Then get off the scale. An hour later, get back on and weigh yourself again. Chances are, you will have two different weights, but it's highly unlikely that your weight actually changed in an hour. Instead, the difference in results is due to random chance, which is a function of how accurately you can measure something. If something is hard to measure, random chance will mean that several measurements of the same thing are likely to give different results. Your weight did not really change; instead, your bathroom scale had difficulty measuring your weight accurately and came up with two different measures of the same thing.

Inferential Statistics

Inferential statistics are used to make generalizations from samples to the population from which the sample was taken. The tests used in inferential statistics, which are based on probability theory, also can serve to determine differences between groups. At least two tests, the t-test and the chi-square test, are useful for pharmacists to know and understand.

The t-test is used to test the differences between two means. If you wanted to know whether the average number of blood glucose monitorings per day for those people who used insulin differed from those who did not use insulin, you would do a t-test. In statistical testing, by convention, you assume that there is no difference between the two results. This is called the null hypothesis. To test the null hypothesis—that there is no significant difference between the two means—you apply the t-test. If the t-test statistic is less than the critical t-value, you fail to reject the null hypothesis and conclude that the means are not different. The critical t-value is a value in statistical tables that is identified by knowing the degrees of freedom of your test, with alpha set at 0.05. (Alpha, which you always set in advance, is the level of significance required.) The formula for calculating degrees of freedom when you have two groups is generally $n_1 + n_2 - 2$, where n_1 is the number of cases in Group 1 and n_2 is the number of cases in Group 2. This formula is appropriate for sample sizes larger than 30 when the number of cases in each group is similar.

The formula for the t-test statistic is shown below.[37] Y_1 is the mean in Group 1 and Y_2 is the mean in Group 2. S_1^2 is the variance in Group 1, S_2^2 is the variance in Group 2, and n is the number of cases.

$$t_s = \frac{Y_1 - Y_2}{\sqrt{1/n\,(s_1^2 + s_2^2)}}$$

In Table 9-4 are examples of statistical tests from another data set. You can see that the t-test statistic for age is 1.1 with 357 degrees of freedom. Statistical tables indicate that the p-value for this t-test statistic is 0.27.

A p-value is similar to alpha except that it is calculated from the data and is not determined in advance. For this set of data, p is calculated to be 0.27. You would fail to reject the null hypothesis and conclude that the means are not different. In most statistical testing, an alpha of 0.05 is considered to be the standard level of significance. If you had calculated that p was less than 0.05, then you would reject the null hypothesis and conclude with 95% confidence that the difference between the means is statistically significant.

Table 9-4. Example of Reporting Statistics

	Treatment (n = 159)	Control (n = 204)	Test Statistic, degrees of freedom, p-value
Age	73.89 ± 6.09	73.18 ± 6.11	$t = -1.1$, 357 df,* p = 0.27
Gender (% male)	36.5%	30.4%	$\chi 2 = 1.1$, 1df, p = 0.27
Income			$\chi 2 = 1.2$, 3df, p = 0.74
< $20,000	40%	40%	
$20,000-$39,000	40%	43%	
$40,000-$59,000	11%	11%	
$60,000 or greater	8%	5%	

*357 degrees of freedom suggests that not all subjects answered this question. Otherwise, there would have been 361 degrees of freedom (159 + 204) – 2 = 361.

Note: χ is the Greek symbol for chi.

Pharmacists should also be familiar with the chi-square test, which is used to determine whether the frequency distribution (i.e., proportion) between two or more groups is different. This test is actually a comparison of observed versus expected frequencies, and is based on a null hypothesis that there is no relationship between variables and the groups in the total population. Table 9-5 shows the number of people in a study who received follow-up phone calls and whether they are compliant with their medications. These are observed data.

You use Table 9-5 (the data you observed) to calculate Table 9-6 (the data that would be expected). The expected values are calculated as (Total number observed in each row ÷ Grand total) × (Total number observed in each column). For example, the data show that 23 patients who were compliant with therapy also received follow-up phone calls. This is the observed result. You calculate the expected result as the row total (55) divided by the grand total (100) and multiplied by the column total (60). As shown in Table 9-6, you would expect to see 33 compliant patients who also received a follow-up phone call, not the 23 that you actually observed.

Table 9-5. Observed Data Regarding Follow-up Calls

Observed		Received Follow-up Phone Calls		
		Yes	No	Totals
	Yes	23	32	55
Compliance	No	37	8	45
	Totals	60	40	100

Table 9-6. Expected Value of Each Cell

Expected		Received Follow-up Phone Calls		
		Yes	No	Totals
	Yes	55/100 × 60 = 33	55/100 × 40 = 22	55
Compliance	No	45/100 × 60 = 27	45/100 × 40 = 18	45
	Totals	60	40	100

Then, you calculate a chi-square value for each cell using the formula (Observed − Expected)^2 ÷ Expected. For example, the chi-square value for the cell of compliant patients who received follow-up phone calls would be $(23 − 33)^2 ÷ 33 = 3.03$. You do the same calculation for the remaining cells in Table 9-7 and add them together. If the total exceeds the critical value of chi square, you reject the null hypothesis and conclude that the two groups are different.

Table 9-7. Chi-Square Values

Cell chi square = (observed − expected)²/ expected		Received Follow-up Phone Calls		
		Yes	No	Totals
	Yes	3.03	4.54	7.57
Compliance	No	3.70	5.55	9.25

In this example, the chi-square statistic (the sum of the chi-square cells) is calculated to be 16.82 (3.03 + 4.54 + 3.70 + 5.55 = 16.82). Use the standard alpha of 0.05 to be 95% sure that rejecting the null hypothesis is correct and that the difference we measured is significant. You have 1 degree of freedom (calculated as r − 1 × c − 1, where r is the number of rows in the table [2] and c is the number of columns [2]). A statistics table shows that the critical value of chi square is 3.841 for an alpha of 0.05 and 1 degree of freedom. Since the calculated chi square (16.82) exceeds the critical value (3.841), you would reject the null hypothesis and conclude that patients who received follow-up phone calls had significantly different rates of compliance compared to those who did not receive follow-up phone calls. Unfortunately, this tells you that those patients who received follow-up phone calls were actually *less* compliant.

In other cases, the chi square tells you that you must fail to reject the null hypothesis. Table 9-4 also shows the proportion of male patients in the study as well as the proportion of patients distributed into each income group. If you were to perform chi-square tests for gender and income distribution, you would find in each case that the chi square you calculated did not exceed the critical value using an alpha of 0.05. In other words, you would fail to reject the null hypothesis and be 95% sure (1 − alpha) that gender and income distribution are not significantly different from the treatment and control groups.

Data analysis can seem like a daunting task, but it's necessary to prevent you from reaching incorrect conclusions. Suppose, for example, that you conducted a small test of a new patient care program to see how it works before fully incorporating it into your practice. Now suppose that 50% of patients in the new program group had a good outcome but only 40% of patients you treated the old way had a good outcome. Do you decide to move ahead and incorporate the new program into your practice? Just looking at the raw data, you'd say "yes." But what if the 10% difference between groups was just a random variation in the numbers? Then you might put a new program into effect and find that it doesn't create the results you want. Statistical testing, no matter how tedious it appears, allows you to make an informed decision about what your data mean so you don't have to accept the data at face value. Basically, you just need to know:

+ The level of measurement you have for your variables.
+ The kind of data that will best answer your question.
+ How accurately you can measure your variables of interest.
+ How big a difference you need to see before you feel the difference is important.
+ What you are trying to compare.
+ How many groups you have.

This information is sufficient to direct you towards the proper statistical test. For a more complete description of these tests you can refer to a number of research-oriented books. [35]

Use of Consultants

Several resources are available if you have research questions, projects that you want evaluated, or complicated statistics to be calculated. Hiring a private company may be expensive but is likely to provide timely data. You could use the Yellow Pages, Internet, or other directories to find business, economic, and financial consultants likely to have the statistical background to help you. You could also contact a researcher at a university. Many researchers would be willing to answer the research questions of motivated pharmacists, and although their services are unlikely to be free, they will probably be less costly than those of a private company. Another option is to contact local pharmacy associations. Staff at these organizations are often familiar with data management and analysis and they may be able to assist you.

One note of caution: contact whoever you choose to help you *before* designing your study and deciding which data to collect. Experienced statisticians have endless horror stories of people waving floppy disks at them and pleading for help, only to discover that the data are too fouled up to be interpretable. Meeting with a statistical expert in advance can be both faster and cheaper than looking for assistance when it's too late to make changes in your study design.

Research and Publication

If you have research analyses that represent new information, or findings that confirm or refute previous information, it is important that you publish your work. In addition to workshops, books, and articles that can help you with this process, you may be able to get assistance from experienced university researchers. Here are some tips on how to write up your research for publication:

1. Go to a medical library and find journals that publish pharmacy practice research studies. The *Journal of the American Pharmaceutical Association*,

The *American Journal of Health-System Pharmacy*, or *The Annals of Pharmacotherapy* are excellent examples. Read a few articles in each and note what kinds of studies each publishes. Most follow a consistent format that you can use as a guide.

2. After you find a journal that is likely to be interested in the kind of study you have done, get a copy of its "Instructions for Authors," usually available on the journal's Web site or by mail or fax from the organization that publishes the journal. Follow these instructions exactly. Failing to submit an article in the required form guarantees that it will be rejected, even if it represents important new work.

3. Most journal editors will be glad to give you broad guidance about preparing an article for publication. Don't expect editors to help you write your article, but don't be afraid to contact them and ask for advice. They *want* to see prospective authors succeed. After all, without authors, there would be no need for editors.

Appendix: Example of Patient Study Information Sheet

Health Care Outcomes of Senior Albertans after the Provision of Pharmaceutical Care

Patient Study Information Sheet – Group A
Principal Investigator: Roger Research, PharmD
Co-investigators: Sally Study, MD
                     Nick Numbercruncher, PhD

Background

Your pharmacists at STUDY PHARMACY NAME have agreed to take part in a study to see how they can help you with your medications and what impact their activities have. Typically, your pharmacist provides you with medications and checks to be sure the dose and number of times you take the drug are okay. Your pharmacist may also check all your drugs to make sure that none will interact and cause you problems. Your pharmacist may answer questions about your medicines. However, your pharmacist believes that he/she can do more to help you because of the number of drugs you are taking. Your pharmacist also believes that you can help him/her and your physician identify the best medicines for you.

Purpose

You are being asked to participate in a research study to compare the care you get from your pharmacist with the care other patients get from their pharmacists. We are doing this study because medicine use by seniors may not be the best it can be and we want to see if pharmacists can help improve medicine use among seniors.

Procedures

Participation in this study will involve:

a) Completing four telephone interviews over a 15-month period. Each interview will take about 20 minutes to complete.
b) Completing a diary over the study period that states the reason and dates of nonprescription drug purchases, physician office visits, hospitalizations, and other health care services.
c) Providing permission to use your Alberta Health identification number and your pharmacy records so that we can quantify use of the health care system.

Your physician will be notified that you are participating in the study.

Appendix: Example of Patient Study Sheet, continued

Possible Benefits

The possible benefits to you for participating in this study are that you may improve your quality of life because drug-related problems are controlled. You may gain confidence in managing your medications and associated problems. You may learn more about your medications, their desired effects, and how to monitor your reaction to the medications. You will probably be able to provide more clear information about your reaction to your medications for your physician, pharmacist, or other caregivers.

Possible Risks

There could be side effects from your medications that are impossible to anticipate. It is important that you immediately notify your physician or pharmacist or one of the individuals listed at the end of this information sheet if you experience any unusual symptoms or have any concerns.

Confidentiality

Personal records relating to this study will be kept confidential. Any report published as a result of this study will not identify you by name.

We would be grateful if you would help carry out this 18-month project. If, for whatever reason, you want to stop being in the study, you are free to withdraw at any time. Your current level of pharmacy care will not be affected in any way. If the study is not undertaken or if it is discontinued at any time, the quality of your pharmacy care will not be affected. If any knowledge gained from this or any other study becomes available that could influence your decision to continue in the study, you will be promptly informed.

Please contact any of the individuals identified below if you have any questions or concerns:

Roger Research, PharmD, Assistant Professor
College of Pharmacy and Health Sciences
Phone: 555-123-4567

Sally Study, MD, Assistant Professor
College of Pharmacy and Health Sciences
Phone: 555-234-5678

Nick Numbercruncher, PhD, Assistant Professor
College of Pharmacy and Health Sciences
Phone: 555-345-6789

References

1. Manasse HR. Medication use in an imperfect world: drug misadventuring as an issue of public policy, part 1. *Am J Hosp Pharm.* 1989;46:929-44.

2. Manasse HR. Medication use in an imperfect world: drug misadventuring as an issue of public policy, part 2. *Am J Hosp Pharm.* 1989;46:1141-52.

3. Committee on Quality of Health Care in America, Institute of Medicine; Kohn LT, Corrigan JM, Donaldson MS, eds. *To Err is Human: Building a Safer Health System.* Washington, DC: National Academy Press; 2000.

4. Hatoum HT, Akhras K. 1993 bibliography: a 32-year literature review on the value and acceptance of ambulatory care provided by pharmacists. *Ann Pharmacother.* 1993;27:1106-19.

5. Rupp MT. Value of community pharmacists' interventions to correct prescribing errors. *Ann Pharmacother.* 1992;26:1580-4.

6. Morrison A, Wertheimer AI. Evaluation of studies investigating the effectiveness of pharmacists' clinical services. *Am J Health-Syst Pharm.* 2001;58:569-77.

7. Munroe WP, Kunz K, Dalmady-Israel C, et al. Economic evaluation of pharmacist involvement in disease management in a community pharmacy setting. *Clin Ther.* 1997;19:113-23.

8. Coast-Senior EA, Kroner BA, Kelley CL, et al. Management of patients with type 2 diabetes by pharmacists in primary care clinics. *Ann Pharmacother.* 1998;32:636-41.

9. Knight W. Quality of care. In: *Managed Care: What It Is and How It Works.* Gaithersburg, MD: Aspen Publishers, Inc; 1998.

10. Hepler CD, Strand LM. Opportunities and responsibilities in pharmaceutical care. *Am J Hosp Pharm.* 1990;47:533-43.

11. McDowell I, Newell C. General health status and quality of life. In: *Measuring Health, a Guide to Rating Scales and Questionnaires.* 2nd ed. New York: Oxford University Press; 1996; chap 9.

12. Quality Metric, Inc: SF-36. Available at: http://www.qmetric.com/innohome/insf36.shtml. Accessed February 2, 2002.

13. Patrick DL, Chiang YP. Health outcomes methodologies symposium proceedings. *Med Care.* 2000;38(9)(suppl II):14-25.

14. Adamcik BA. The consumers of health care. In: Fincham JE, Wertheimer AI, eds. *Pharmacy and the U.S. Health Care System.* 2nd ed. New York: Haworth Press, Inc; 1998; chap 14.

15. Glanz K, Lewis FD, Rimer BK, eds. *Health Behavior and Health Education: Theory, Research and Practice.* 2nd ed. San Francisco: Jossey-Bass Publishers, 1997.

16. Morisky DE, Green LW, Levine DM. Concurrent and predictive validity of a self-reported measure of medication adherence. *Med Care.* 1986;24:67-74.

17. Steiner JF, Koepsell TD, Fihn SD, et al. A general method of compliance assessment using centralized pharmacy records. *Med Care.* 1988;26:814-23.

18. Maddigan SL. *Predictors of Success, Failure and Errors in a Geriatric Self-Medication Program: A Retrospective Chart Review.* Edmonton, Alberta, Canada:

University of Alberta; 2000. Thesis.

19. Botelho RJ, Dudrak R. Home assessment of adherence to long-term medication in the elderly. *J Fam Pract.* 1992;25:61-5.

20. Coons SJ, Sheahan SL, Martin SS, et al. Predictors of medication noncompliance in a sample of older adults. *Clin Ther.* 1994;16:110-17.

21. Larrat EP, Taubman AH, Willey CW. Compliance-related problems in the ambulatory population. *American Pharmacy.* 1990;NS30:82-7.

22. Ryan AA. Medication compliance and older people: a review of the literature. *Int J Nurs Stud.* 1999;36:153-62.

23. Allen SM, Mor V. The prevalence and consequences of unmet need: contrasts between older and younger adults with disability. *Med Care.* 1997;35:1132-48.

24. Campbell VA, Crews JE, Moriarty DG, et al. Surveillance for sensory impairment, activity limitation, and health-related quality of life among older adults: United States, 1993–1997. *MMWR.* 1999;48(SS8):131-56.

25. MacKeigan LD, Larson LN. Development and validation of an instrument to measure patient satisfaction with pharmacy services. *Med Care.* 1989;27:522-36.

26. Johnson JA, Coons SJ, Hays RD. The structure of satisfaction with pharmacy services. *Med Care.* 1998;36:244-50.

27. Ware JE, Snyder MK, Wright WR, et al. Defining and measuring patient satisfaction with medical care. *Evaluation and Program Planning.* 1983;6:247-63.

28. Johnson KA, Parker JP, McCombs JS, et al. The Kaiser Permanente/USC Patient Consultation Study: patient satisfaction with pharmaceutical services. *Am J Health Syst Pharm.* 1998;55:2621-9.

29. Larson LN, Rovers JP, MacKeigan LD. Patient satisfaction with pharmaceutical care: update of a validated instrument. *J Am Pharm Assoc.* 2002;42:44-50.

30. Lohr K. How do we measure quality. *Health Aff.* 1996;16(3)(May/June):22-25.

31. Farris KB, Kirking DM. Assessing the quality of pharmaceutical care II. Application of concepts of quality assessment from medical care. *Ann Pharmacother.* 1993;27:215-23.

32. Farris KB, Kirking DM. Assessing the quality of pharmaceutical care I. One perspective of quality. *Ann Pharmacother.* 1993;27:68-73.

33. Motheral BR, Schafermeyer KW. Managed health care. In: McCarthy RI, Schafermeyer KW, eds. *Introduction to Health Care Delivery, A Primer for Pharmacists.* Gaithersburg, MD: Aspen Publishers, Inc; 2001.

34. Cal. Bus. & Prof Code § 4125 (West Supp. 2002).

35. Babbie E. *The Practice of Social Research.* 9th ed. Stamford, CT: Wadsworth Thomson Learning; 2001.

36. Lo B. Addressing ethical issues. In: Hulley SB, Cummings SR, et al., eds. *Designing Clinical Research: An Epidemiologic Approach.* 2nd ed. Philadelphia: Lippincott Williams & Wilkins; 2001.

37. Sokal RR, Rohlf FJ. *Biometry.* 2nd ed. New York: Freeman and Company; 1981.

Chapter 10
CONTINUOUS QUALITY IMPROVEMENT
Susan J. Skledar

Few issues in health care have become more important and more widely discussed than quality of care. Although pharmacists, like other health care providers, probably believe that they provide high-quality care, they usually do not have much data to support what are basically just their opinions. Payers have a vested interest in ensuring that the providers in their networks give the best care possible. To that end, they are increasingly tying reimbursement to the quality of care provided. Consequently, for your patient care programs to be successful you must be able to demonstrate both the quality of your care and any improvements in your care.

This chapter describes in detail how you can develop your own quality assurance programs. Some of the concepts in this chapter draw on material from other chapters, such as developing a vision and philosophy of practice (Chapter 2), creating interdisciplinary teams (Chapter 3), and collecting and interpreting patient outcomes data (Chapter 9).

A Historical Perspective

There is a wealth of published literature on quality improvement in health care. You can find information as far back as the mid 1800s on gathering and analyzing hospital statistics. Efforts to evaluate quality of work emerged in the 1900s, including health care quality measurement efforts pioneered by Ernest A. Codman.[1] In the early 1900s the American College of Surgeons (ACS) engineered the first standardized approach to monitoring hospitals and providing accreditation. In the 1950s, the ACS merged with the American College of Physicians, American Hospital Association, American Medical Association, and Canadian Medical Association to form the Joint Commission on Accreditation of Hospitals (JCAH, now the Joint Commission on Accreditation of Healthcare Organizations, or JCAHO). The intent of the JCAH was to provide a set of standards for institutions to attain voluntarily. JCAH requirements began with review of medical care and the medical record. They expanded over the 1950s to include standards for other disciplines, including infection control and pharmacy.

As Medicare evolved in the 1960s, hospitals had to maintain JCAH standards of care to participate. In the 1970s, standards became more specific for patient care and ancillary departments, and drug use evaluation by pharmacy and therapeutics review became mandatory. In the late 1970s, a standard was created that required institution-wide quality assurance pro-grams to be adopted and implemented. This requirement led many institutions into the fold of continuous quality improvement (CQI). Systematic models have been adopted to apply CQI to everyday philosophy and practice.

The Pareto Principle

"In any series of elements to be controlled, a selected, small fraction, in terms of the number of elements, always accounts for a large fraction in terms of effect."

—Vilfredo Pareto (1848-1923)

Source: Erickson SM. Management Tools for Everyone: Twenty Techniques. New York: Petrocelli Books, Inc; 1981.

Table 10-1 lists the developers of key CQI principles, including Codman and Joseph M. Juran, seen by many as the "father" of quality.[2] Juran is best known for authoring what is considered the standard reference tool for quality control, *Juran's Quality Handbook*,[3] as well as other key references for quality improvement and the theory of quality management.[4] In the late 1930s, Juran conceptualized the "Pareto Principle"[5] (see box above). Many leaders and administrators rely on this principle today to help focus improvement efforts on the problem that will make the most impact if solved. Juran created many tools for quality improvement teaching, including seminars, video training programs, and reference materials. He is also the expert who added the human perspective to the statistical roots of quality to create what is now termed "Total Quality Management."[2]

Table 10-1. Continuous Quality Improvement Experts

Expert	Era	Pioneer Work
E. A. Codman	1900s	Quality assessment in health care
W. Shewart	1920s	Statistical process control charts Plan-Do-Check-Act cycle
J. M. Juran	1930s	Pareto principle Theory of Quality Management
W. E. Deming	1950s (Japan) 1980s (U.S.)	Fourteen Points Seven Deadly Diseases
A. Donabedian	1960s	Structure-process-outcome Seven Pillars of Quality

Walter Shewart, a statistician, is best known for the statistical process control (SPC) chart. The SPC chart can help detect process variation over time and is a tool for monitoring the ongoing stability of a process. Shewart designed rules for determining when a process is stable or under control, and when it should be acted upon.[6,7] He is also known for developing the Plan-Do-Check-Act (PDCA) cycle, also called the Plan-Do-Study-Act (PDSA) cycle.[6,8] This cycle provides a model that allows you to plan for changes in your project and establish criteria to monitor and measure improvement. Within established time frames you plan, implement or test, evaluate impact, and continually refine or expand the project.

W. Edwards Deming worked with the Japanese to rebuild their society after World War II. He used concepts he learned from his colleague, Shewart, to educate the Japanese about expanding statistical improvement methods to quality work, evaluating consumer needs, and anticipating what the future will respond to. His CQI philosophy, now adopted by many U.S. corporations, promotes continual improvement within aspects of an organization's work and stresses the importance of structuring the work environment to support continual improvement.[7,9] According to Deming's approach, opportunities for improvement should be defined, potential causes of the problem identified, and actions taken to eliminate the causes of problems. Deming's teachings are exemplified in his Fourteen Points,[10] which are meant to transform the philosophy of management to incorporate constant improvement of processes (see box below). As these points were adopted, Deming identified a series of barriers to reform, called The Seven Deadly Diseases"[10] (see sidebar on page 220).

 Deming's 14 Points

Point 1: Create constancy of purpose toward product and service improvement. Be competitive, provide jobs, and stay in business.

Point 2: Adopt a new philosophy. Mistakes and negativity are unacceptable.

Point 3: Cease dependence on mass inspection. Build quality into the process in the first place.

Point 4: End the practice of awarding business on price tag alone.

Point 5: Improve constantly and forever the system of production and service.

Point 6: Institute training.

Point 7: Institute leadership.

Point 8: Drive out fear.

Point 9: Break down barriers between staff areas.

Point 10: Eliminate slogans, exhortations, and targets for the workforce.

Point 11: Eliminate numerical quotas.

Point 12: Remove barriers to pride of workmanship.

Point 13: Institute a vigorous program of education and retraining.

Point 14: Take action to accomplish the transformation.

Avedis Donabedian is credited with having significant impact on the application of quality principles to health care.[11] Donabedian was the first to identify the structure-process-outcome (SPO) model and apply it to medical care.[12,13] Structure represents the attributes of a facility and its capacity to provide quality care. Structure influences process—the activities involved in giving and receiving care. Better processes lead to better outcomes, which are effects or results of the processes of care on patient health. According to Donabedian, the links between structure and process as well as between process and outcome must be understood before quality improvement efforts can be undertaken.[13] When examining provision of medical care, Donabedian identified Seven Pillars of Quality that can characterize quality care[14]:

+ Efficacy.
+ Effectiveness.
+ Efficiency.
+ Acceptability.
+ Optimality.
+ Equity.
+ Legitimacy.

Deming's Seven Deadly Diseases

Disease 1: Lack of constancy of purpose.

Disease 2: Emphasis on short-term profits.

Disease 3: Evaluation by performance, merit rating, or annual review of performance.

Disease 4: Mobility of management.

Disease 5: Running a company on visible figures alone.

Disease 6: Excessive medical costs.*

Disease 7: Excessive costs of warranty, fueled by lawyers who work on a contingency fee basis.*

* Apply only to the United States

These pillars can be used differently depending on one's perspective, such as that of an individual or the larger group. For example, a health system would regard efficiency as a good thing that improves quality. Having one nurse care for 12 patients when she used to care for 8 would be an improvement in efficiency as long as the quality of the nurse's care did not drop below some threshold. From the perspective of the patients in those 12 beds, however, they may not be enthusiastic about having less time with the nurse, even though her care is adequate. Donabedian's principles help us understand quality measurement, but there is still much to know.[13]

The Importance of CQI in Pharmacy Practice

In today's practice, which unfolds in a health care atmosphere of rapid and significant change, CQI concepts are useful for helping pharmacy leaders and administrators rethink procedures and services and optimize care. Providing quality care while balancing resource utilization is an important goal as pharmacy practice forges ahead.

CQI, which focuses on constantly improving the quality of systems or processes, provides leaders with a structure for performance improvement. The entire organization should work toward a goal of continuous improvement in quality, as defined by the customer.[15] Although quality is sometimes perceived as subjective, understanding and measuring it objectively is crucial to improving care. In the 1990s the JCAHO shifted to a heavy CQI focus with emphasis on education, performance improvement, multidisciplinary collaboration in patient care, and standard levels of care. Applying CQI principles can improve care and incorporate all the JCAHO focus areas. Understanding CQI principles is essential to designing sound operational and clinical programs, as well as measuring the impact of programs and services.

Developing a Strategy for CQI

CQI is defined as a systematic, organizational approach for continually improving all processes that deliver quality services and products.[6] The pharmacy and administrative leadership as well as the institution or organization must embrace CQI, and its principles must be integrated into all aspects of departmental and organizational operations. A strategic framework must be designed in which the following take place:[6,9]

+ Define quality and an improvement strategy for your organization.
+ Disseminate the definitions and philosophy to all employees.
+ Designate leadership for CQI efforts for the organization.
+ Create a constancy of purpose.
+ Develop and maintain a strong customer and patient focus.
+ Focus on continually improving processes.
+ Use employee teams as forums for problem-solving and planning.
+ Use data-driven methods to identify opportunities for improvement.
+ Communicate results of efforts.

Organizations need to define quality in terms of commitment to improving outcomes, promoting cost-effective care, and meeting or even exceeding customer expectations. Organizational leaders should decide on a performance improvement philosophy as well as the strategy that will be adopted to carry out improvement efforts. Once defined, this philosophy and strategy must be disseminated to all members of the organization, including leadership and staff. A philosophy cannot be embraced if it is not understood by employees. If truly understood, the philosophy becomes a normal part of problem-solving and of planning and evaluating new services. Integral to this is support from all members of the organization.

Oversight, Customers, and Systematic Processes

Typically, a committee or council is designated to oversee organizational quality efforts. Individual departments or clinical services within organizations often have their own self-directed subcommittees or work groups to identify, develop, implement, and evaluate services and programs. These departments should use a defined system to communicate the results of successful improvement efforts and to suggest opportunities for further study to the larger body. All function teams should use the same philosophy and strategy for improvement. If the CQI strategy is well defined and grounded in the literature, you can compare organizational improvement efforts to those of other similar organizations. A constancy of purpose should underscore all improvement efforts. It is important that all members of the organization understand the philosophy of the organization as well as the CQI strategy and how it relates to their everyday work.

You must focus your improvement efforts on customers, both internal and external.[6] Internal customers can be colleagues, coworkers, other departments, and any other groups that you interface with to complete your work. External customers are best defined as the "end users"; that is, the final recipients of the service or product you are providing.[6] It has been stated that customers will pay more for better quality, and that customer loyalty is maintained when quality is continually improving.[16] Pharmacists' ultimate customer is the patient, but there are also many other customers who receive direct or indirect output of pharmaceutical care services, such as physicians, nurses, students, and payers.

Organizations must continually improve processes, services, and performance and should integrate the quality improvement philosophy into all aspects of work. You should never think that current levels of service or performance are sufficient for the future. Try to anticipate the expectations of the future and strive to meet, or better yet, exceed them.

It's important to have a systematic approach to identifying processes for improvement and to improve those processes using streamlined procedures. The PDCA cycle[6,8] mentioned on page 218 is one such approach to improving processes. Its application to performance improvement will be discussed later in the chapter.

Employee Work Teams

Employee work teams are the best forum for problem-solving and for planning successful improvement efforts. Effective problem-solving needs people (teams), structure, data, and tools. Participation should be encouraged and mentored. Teams, which must be multidisciplinary, are responsible for:

+ Identifying opportunities for improvement.
+ Analyzing causes of problems.
+ Discussing improvement strategies.
+ Educating practitioners.

For teams to be effective they need a mission or objectives that are clearly stated, as well as defined responsibilities and deadlines. The team should have open communication channels, be able to exchange ideas freely, and be focused on the target or expected result. Strong leadership of the team is essential, and as the project unfolds, findings and action steps must be communicated thoroughly to all team members and/or the team's customers. The team's decisions and conclusions should be based on objective findings—either evidence in the literature or internally analyzed data.

People should be encouraged to take part in the teams and team members should not feel threatened or embarrassed by engaging in active discussion. At the same time, everyone must understand that results are the goal; they all want the same positive outcome at the end. Improvement efforts must be clearly communicated and recognized both within and beyond the team. Often, this ignites future improvement efforts or helps provide a template for new projects.

Data-Driven Processes

Identifying opportunities for improving processes and for reporting progress and results should be data-driven.[7] Displaying information graphically can help you analyze the current process and address the root cause of problems.[5] Having a sophisticated information system lets you gather and analyze data efficiently, but you can do the work manually as long as you understand that a larger time commitment will be needed. Data for improvement projects can be abstracted from clinical information systems, billing records, archived data, questionnaires, insurance records, and admission databases. Displaying the data in a systematic way, using graphics such as SPC charts[6,7] or Pareto charts[5] helps you use consistent improvement approaches and allows for uniform interpretation of findings. (See page 229 for a sample SPC chart and page 232 for a sample Pareto chart.) Applying SPC charts, Pareto charts, and similar tools to results data can quickly point out successful, stable efforts, showcase opportunities for improvement, or highlight the need for re-education.

Planning Your CQI Project (PLAN)

A set of three questions forms the basis for all quality improvement efforts:[17,18]

+ What are we trying to accomplish?
+ How will we know that a change is an improvement?
+ What changes can we make that will result in an improvement?

The first question attempts to define the project's aim. Depending on the formality of the project, you should draft a goal or mission statement and objectives. Identify a specific, measurable goal for your project as well as a specific time frame in which to reach your goal. To answer the second question you must know the baseline practice and the desired level of change, and you must have a system in place to measure the impact of the changed or improved process. Flow charts and brainstorming are two useful tools for understanding current processes and determining changes that you will make to answer the third question.

For example, a way to measure whether a change to a different method of doing a diagnostic test is an improvement would be to measure how accurate the test is in a sample number of patients or to survey patients about their comfort level with the test. You can use a series of CQI tools and techniques to identify root causes of problems, prioritize them, and figure out which changes will result in the most improvement. These tools and techniques are outlined in Table 10-2 on the PDCA cycle and further detailed in the steps that follow.

Table 10-2. Stepwise Approach to Applying the PDCA Cycle

Phase of the PDCA Cycle	Actions
PLAN	Define the problem
	Create a multidisciplinary team to address the issue
	Define key quality indicators
	Analyze baseline data
	Review current practices
	Perform root cause analysis
	Create action plan for change
DO	Implement recommendations for change
CHECK	Reassess indicators and demonstrate improvement
ACT	Design future plans and establish system for ongoing monitoring

Step 1: Define the Problem

To define your problem you must have a data-driven need for improvement. Information that is leading your group to solve the problem could be, for example, multiple reports of adverse reactions related to a particular drug. State the problem in relation to organizational performance and be sure it is a measurable problem, not an anecdotal report of concern. Distill the problem into manageable pieces so your project is not too complex to achieve results. For example, asking why postoperative infections happen in your institution would be an enormous undertaking because it involves evaluating risk for various types of surgeries, underlying diseases of the patients, variability in surgical technique across all your surgeons, and

Figure 10-1. Sample Quality Indicator

Indicator objective:
This indicator will measure compliance with recommendations for timing of administration of presurgical antimicrobial doses. The optimal time for administering presurgical antimicrobial doses to best prevent postsurgical wound infection is within 120 minutes prior to surgical incision[19]
Numerator:
Number of patients receiving presurgical antimicrobial doses within 120 minutes prior to surgical incision
Denominator:
Number of patients audited undergoing the specified surgical procedure
Goal: audit 150 patients per month
Study population:
Total knee replacement (N=50)
Coronary artery bypass graft (N=50)
Craniectomy (N=50)
Source of data:
Patient anesthesia record
Pharmacy medication dispensing data
Operating room management information system
Threshold for results:
≥ 90% of presurgical antimicrobial doses are administered within 120 minutes prior to surgical incision
Frequency of reporting:
Audit surgeries monthly and report results quarterly
Responsibility for reporting:
Pharmacy will audit patients monthly and prepare report
Reporting structure:
Data will be reported to Pharmacy Quality Improvement Committee, Surgical Services Committee, and Institution Quality Improvement Council

multiple other factors. A more manageable statement of the problem could be that you wish to evaluate ways of ensuring that presurgical doses of prophylactic antibiotics are delivered to the operating room in time for administration within 120 minutes before surgery, as shown in Figure 10-1.

The statement of the problem should never imply the cause or solution and should not suggest blame in any way. When defining the problem, evidence from the literature is the best support for why a topic is being examined. National indicators are put forth by such groups as JCAHO and the Agency for Healthcare Research and Quality (AHRQ). The American Diabetes Association, the American Pain Society, and other national organizations publish standards of care that can be the impetus for CQI projects. You can also benchmark against internal or external standards, focus group information, and customer satisfaction data. Sources of internal information include budget reports, purchasing reports, patient surveys, staff surveys, and brainstorming sessions in which team members suggest possible sources of benchmarking data and share anecdotal reports that may be helpful in defining the problem.

Step 2: Create a Multidisciplinary Team to Address the Issue

The importance of multidisciplinary collaboration on CQI projects cannot be overstated. Interdisciplinary teamwork is key not only in caring for patients or providing products to customers, but also in discovering root causes of problems and potential solutions. If you can identify the chief stakeholders in the process and the expectations of customers it will help keep the project on track and will involve in decision-making anyone with a major investment in the process.

Ideally, you can assemble a team of experts and assign each person responsibilities, such as leading the project, recording the minutes, or analyzing the data. It is also a good idea to enlist administrative support for your project, both within your department and at higher levels if needed. If your project involves defining the uses of a particular drug or determining approaches to treating a disease, a preliminary review of patient charts or computerized records may suggest who the major players should be on your project team. For instance, if existing information suggests that a group of physicians who practice together accounts for 75% of the use of a given drug, inviting one of them to join your group will probably be useful.

Time is at a premium in today's practice environment and a decision to hold meetings to plan your project should not be made lightly. The team leader needs to ensure that meetings will be productive. Nevertheless, some formal team meetings will be necessary to help team members feel comfortable with the project and encourage them to bring up issues, discuss progress, or identify obstacles. Alternatives to team meetings are exchanging information by phone or e-mail. The editing function on word processing programs is also useful for making comments and suggesting changes to other team members.

Step 3: Define Key Quality Indicators

You must select appropriate indicators to measure the extent of your problem and the impact of changes made to improve it. Indicators are rate-based measures. They should specify numerator and denominator, source of data, reporting frequency and structure, study population, and necessary thresholds. If you look at Figure 10-1, a sample quality indicator for analyzing the timing of presurgical antimicrobials in accordance with published literature,[19] you can see these concepts applied.

It is important that you audit a representative sample to obtain your results. Typically, if performing a chart review, a good sample size is 50 charts. If auditing a large number of occurrences, aim to evaluate 10% to 20% of the total occurrences to get a representative sample. It is a good idea to have more than one quality indicator for your project, especially if the indicator is financial. Outcome indicators can be economic (cost savings, cost avoidance), clinical (reduced bleeding episodes, reduced renal toxicity), humanistic (pain control, quality of life), or process outcomes (compliance, number of consults obtained). A combination approach of at least two outcomes is best.

Step 4: Analyze Baseline Data

Current practices—the current "state of affairs"—must be analyzed to give you an understanding of the problem's extent. A CQI project is a data-driven process, so you have to evaluate baseline practices to know the magnitude of your problem, confirm your multidisciplinary team members, and potentially justify resources needed for solutions. Measure the indicator data at several points in time to demonstrate that the occurrence is not a one-time event, but an ongoing problem, before you change your process. A common mistake is to display the information as a single data point rather than using bar charts, run charts, SPC charts, or other graphics.

A bar chart is useful for displaying data when you have two or fewer data points (see Figure 10-2). A run chart monitors a process over time for specific trends or patterns[6] (see Figure 10-3). An SPC chart monitors a process over time by studying variation and the source of variation[6] (see Figure 10-4). You can also display data collected over time using a histogram,[6] which represents the data as frequency distribution; for example, a bell-shaped curve showing a range of exam scores.

The SPC chart provides the most comprehensive data display because it helps identify variation in your process, shows stability, and helps sort out special causes of variation versus common, expected causes.

Figure 10-2. Sample Bar Chart

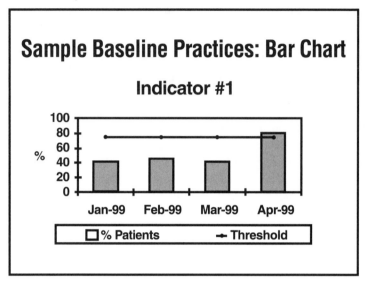

Figure 10-3. Sample Run Chart

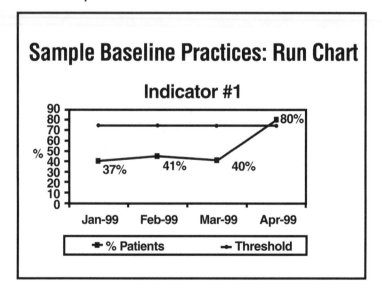

Figure 10-4. Sample Statistical Process Control (SPC) Chart

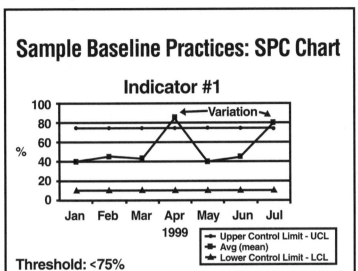

Figure 10-5. Sample Flow Chart

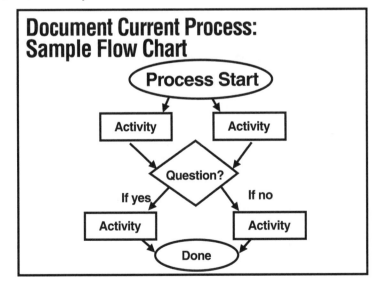

Step 5: Review Current Practices

The most helpful tool in reviewing the current process is the flow chart (see Figure 10-5), which generally uses boxes to show activity steps, diamonds to show decisions, and ovals to show the start and finish of the process. After your multidisciplinary team gathers to discuss the current practice, they should display it as a flow chart, showing all major decision and action points needed to reach the final outcome. The flow chart can help to show the complexity of a process as well as tasks or procedures that are redundant. Furthermore, the final version can be a source of consensus. A key thing to remember when constructing a flow chart is to map out the real process, not the ideal.[6]

Step 6: Perform Root Cause Analysis

After the problem has been demonstrated and the current process defined, you need to identify the root cause of the problem. Your multidisciplinary group should start this step with a brainstorming session to generate as many causes of the problem as possible. The group should feel comfortable exchanging information freely and creatively to generate a large number of ideas. Brainstorming can help to escape the "IOPP" problem—inertia of previous practice[20]— and encourage open thinking. Brainstorming sessions can be structured or unstructured.[6] In the structured approach, each team member contributes one idea per turn, without excessive explanation. All ideas are recorded and reviewed at the end to eliminate duplication or unclear suggestions. In the unstructured approach, team members contribute ideas as they occur.

Once all ideas are generated, they need to be grouped into common categories or major causes. The CQI tool used to do this is known as the cause-and-effect diagram or fishbone diagram,[5-7] also called the Ishihara diagram after its inventor, Kara Ishihara.[5] This diagram helps you list and further explore all the causes identified during the brainstorming and group them into categories to help find the root cause of the problem. General categories often used for groupings include the "four Ps"—people, policies, procedures, and plant—and the "four Ms"—machines, methods, materials, and man.[6] The diagram is flexible because many variations to these categories—or headings for the major causes or "bones"—are possible. Figure 10-6 shows the basic framework for the fishbone diagram, with materials, man, methods, and machine as the major cause categories. To create a fishbone diagram you place the problem you are trying to solve in the box at the right. Then you put under the major "bone" headings on the diagram the problem causes that emerge as you brainstorm. Deeper, minor causes should be drilled down as extensions from the major headings. Once all your causes are diagrammed, you are ready to prioritize opportunities for improvement.

Figure 10-6. Sample Ishihara Diagram

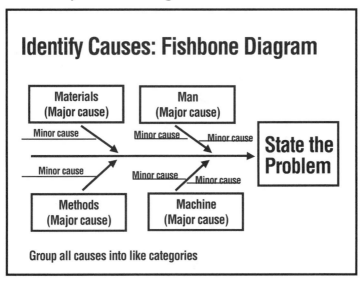

Make sure all causes from your fishbone diagram are grouped into like categories. Then, to rank them, use the Pareto chart.[5,6] As noted earlier, the Pareto principle was operationalized in the 1930s by Joseph M. Juran, who concluded that a vital few members of a group account for most of the total effect. In other words, you should focus your efforts on identifying the "vital few and the trivial many."[3,4,7] Pareto charts (see Figure 10-7) help the team focus on the causes that can affect the problem the most. They are frequency distribution graphs that rank specific causes in order of frequency of occurrence, from highest to lowest. Often, cumulative percentage is graphed on the right axis to display total effect. If you can address the root cause of the problem—the tallest bar on the Pareto chart—you can reduce or even eliminate the problem.

Step 7: Create an Action Plan for Change

This is the last step in the "PLAN" phase of the PDCA cycle. Now your goal is improvement in the process. You must clearly state how you will make changes to solve the problem and base your recommendations for improvement on data from the literature or demonstrated successful processes from other benchmarks or expertise. It's important to obtain any necessary formal approvals for your recommendations from such groups as the Pharmacy and Therapeutics (P&T) Committee, Nursing/Pharmacy Committee, or Medical Executive Committee. Administrative support is essential in facilitating projects and implementing them.

Figure 10-7. Sample Pareto Chart

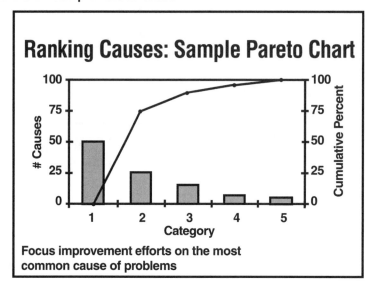

Consider designing your action plan in the form of a pilot project so problems can be smoothed out before the project is expanded. Often, a pilot or test of a new project eases transition. It also allows you to solve problems concurrently, collect detailed data on success, and identify outliers. Multidisciplinary team members can take part in this step of planning and it is also a good idea to identify other staff members to help lead the change. Involvement of front-line staff is especially important in providing a comprehensive quality improvement project.

Implementing Your CQI Project (DO)

The implementation or "do" phase of the CQI project is crucial. Keys to success are defining responsibilities, educating, assessing competency, and adhering to the timetable established by the multidisciplinary team.

Step 8: Implement Recommendations for Change

The multidisciplinary team must typically meet several times to refine and discuss details of the action steps needed to make changes. List the necessary action steps and assign each one to a team member.

Education is the key component of implementation. Members of the multidisciplinary group can help educate practitioners on the new processes. Education should be multidisciplinary—that is, aimed at all practitioners who are in any way involved in the care of patients or in the project. Education should also be multifaceted—a combination approach of written, verbal, and electronic means. Written education may include memoranda, posters, and pocket cards. Verbal education might include training sessions, train-the-trainer meetings, formal seminars, or one-on-one teaching. Electronic means may include e-mail and posting education information on the Internet.

JCAHO standards require assurance of clinical competency for health care staff. This may include assessing staff on their understanding of CQI principles or on their understanding of your current project and its intended outcomes. A timetable for putting the recommended changes in place should be designed and adhered to. The leader of the team is responsible for monitoring progress toward the changes and refocusing group efforts if problems arise.

Studying Your CQI Project (CHECK)

Step 9: Reassess Indicators and Demonstrate Improvement
In this step, you check the results of your pilot or of the change process you have implemented. During Step 3, you designed indicators to measure the program's impact, which included establishing a threshold. Now you measure the outcome data from the implemented changes over time and compare them to established thresholds and pre-implementation data.

As trends begin to emerge from your data analysis, state the results clearly. One effective way to supplement your results statements is to redo your flow chart to show the simplified or amplified process steps you developed. New or changed steps can be made a different color on the flow chart to highlight actions.

You can also graph your post-implementation indicator data to measure impact. If you have enough data points—20 to 25 is considered sufficient[6]—you can calculate upper and lower control limits and a mean value for your indicator data to show stability of the process change over time and to highlight causes of variation. One way to graph this is using an SPC chart, as shown in Figure 10-8. The figure gives the mean of the process, the upper control limit (UCL), and the lower control limit (LCL) and how they change from before to after the process was modified. As you can see in Figure 10-8, the process stabilized after the change was made in August. The mean of the process dropped consistently below the 50% threshold value and the UCL and LCL differences narrowed, indicating less variability in the process.

Figure 10-8. *Sample SPC Chart with Outcome Data*

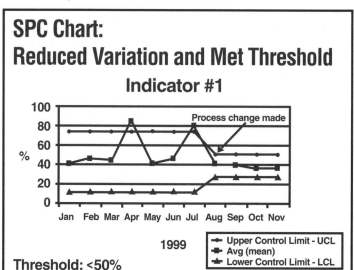

During this step you should evaluate any barriers or obstacles to implementation that have surfaced. Among reasons why the project may not work are:[21]

- Lack of awareness.
- Lack of understanding.
- Information not readily available.
- Lack of confidence in recommendations.
- System inefficiencies.

If the threshold has not been achieved, the multidisciplinary team must look at the improvement process carefully. The improvement cycle may need to be repeated and expansion of the pilot project postponed until improvements can be made. Staff may need to be re-educated or you may have to make minor adjustments to the process. Part of the education process may include giving feedback to the major stakeholders—pharmacists, nurses, physicians, or anyone else affected by the new process. You may need new forms of education, such as increased teaching sessions or mock scenarios.

Determining Course of Action (ACT)

Step 10: Design Future Plans and Establish System for Ongoing Monitoring

At this point, the pilot may be expanding and procedures or services may be standardized. You should evaluate indicators at the same time and select the next process for improvement.

If the threshold was achieved, you move ahead to expand the process and standardize the changes in procedures or services throughout the system. At this time, you should also begin to discuss and identify the next process for improvement and set targets for it. Adding on the next level of improvements when one phase of the project is done is called "cycling." The cycling repeats until improvements are made and sustained or the threshold is exceeded.

Alternatively, if your threshold for the original project was not achieved, you need to make additional improvements in how you are changing the process and keep reassessing your indicators until you reach the threshold.

This final step in the CQI process—also known as "holding the gains" or "checking for backsliding"—is one of the most important. Systems must be set up to monitor compliance and outcomes so improvements and variability are evaluated on an ongoing basis. Such systems allow you to refine processes for maximum efficiency and optimal quality. Among the monitoring mechanisms you might use are periodic team meetings, quarterly assessments, literature reviews, and status reports.

You should establish a reporting schedule for your department and for multidisciplinary committees such as the Quality Improvement Committee, Operations Committee, or P&T Committee. Identify who has responsibility for gathering the data and preparing the report and determine the frequency of reporting. Usually monitoring is more intensive at the start of a CQI project. Once the threshold is reached and sustained, monitoring can be scaled back to monthly or bimonthly. Quarterly or semi-annual review of CQI projects is best to make sure that the project's impact is maintained and to identify special causes of variation that can ignite the CQI cycle again.

Understanding and Interpreting Variability

The statistical process control chart, or SPC (see Figure 10-8), is one of the best CQI tools for illustrating variability within a process or showing that systems are out of control. It is important for departmental CQI leaders to understand these charts so they are used in a meaningful way. In the words of Deming, "proliferation of charts without purpose is to be avoided."[7,22]

In SPC charts, the "x" axis is a time frame and the "y" axis is the measurement. Outcome indicator data are plotted over time against three other variables:

1. The upper control limit (UCL).
2. The lower control limit (LCL).
3. The mean.

The UCL and LCL represent the mean plus or minus three standard deviations. These limits capture 99.74% of variation. Although common causes of variation will always occur, the SPC chart helps to distinguish them from "special" causes. Common causes of variation can only be fixed by changing the system, such as modifying procedures or establishing policies.[7] Common causes are usually system problems rather than problems with individuals, and they may even involve chance occurrence or randomness. Special causes of variation are things like lack of training or malfunctioning equipment, which are usually relatively easy to fix.

The more streamlined your process, the less variation and deviation from the mean. The UCL and LCL will not necessarily correspond with your threshold, though. It is possible to have a stable process that is performing well below or above threshold. Control limits display consistency and stability, not necessarily success. Make note of where your mean value falls with respect to your established objective or threshold. If it does not meet the threshold, you have not achieved the project's goal. Your ultimate aim is a mean that meets the threshold value and that also shows stability and consistency in the process.

There are two types of SPC charts: measurable or variable and counted or attribute charts. Measurable charts are further divided into X-bar and R charts; attribute charts are divided into P charts and C charts.[6,7] Measurable data charts are

℞ Rules for Determining Out-of-Control Processes

A process is out of control if any one of these situations is true:

- One point or more is outside of the upper control limit (UCL) or lower control limit (LCL).
- Seven consecutive points are on one side of the mean.
- Six consecutive points are either increasing or decreasing.
- Fourteen consecutive points alternate up and down.
- Fifteen consecutive points are within one standard deviation.
- Two out of three consecutive points on the same side of the mean are greater than two standard deviations.
- Four out of five consecutive points on the same side of the mean are greater than one standard deviation.

Source: Adapted from Brassard M, Ritter D. *The Memory Jogger II: A Pocket Guide of Tools for Continuous Improvement and Effective Planning.* Salem, NH: GOAL/QPC; 1994.

used to graph data that are infinitely variable such as temperature, cost, or pressure. Counted data charts are used to graph data that are counted in discrete units such as medication errors or adverse drug reaction events.

Measurable data charts are plotted together to show both variation within and between subgroups, whereas counted data charts measure variation between samples. UCL and LCL calculations are made according to formulas for three standard deviations from the mean.

It is best to collect 20 to 25 data points to make a meaningful SPC and assure random data collection. Statistical programs and textbooks are available to help calculate UCL and LCL, depending on which type of data you have.[6] For the best measure of your process's stability, the control limits should not change over time, unless you have made a significant change to your process. If so, use new data after the change to calculate new control limits. The box on page 236 provides rules for determining if your process is out of control.

Summary

Using CQI in project planning is crucial. Ideally, a strategic approach to CQI should be adopted within organizations, and the approach should definitely be embraced by pharmacy leadership to measure program impact. Pharmacists can take a leadership role in organizations, institutions, and the community by setting up the structure, process, and outcomes necessary to develop and implement successful pharmaceutical care programs. Continuously evaluating programs for improvement and attainment of goals will keep pharmacy practice competitive and forward thinking far into the future.

References

1. Reverby S. Stealing the golden eggs: Ernest Armory Colman and science and management of medicine. *Bull Hist Med.* 1981;55:156-71.
2. Six Sigma @ Juran Institute. Available at: http://www.juran.com. Accessed March 9, 2000.
3. Juran JM, Godfrey AB. *Juran's Quality Handbook.* 5th ed. New York: McGraw, Hill; 1999.
4. Juran JM, Godfrey AB, Blanton DA. *Managerial Breakthrough: The Classic Book on Improving Management Performance.* 30th anniversary ed. New York: McGraw-Hill International Book Co; 1995.
5. Erickson SM. *Management Tools for Everyone: Twenty Techniques.* New York: Petrocelli Books, Inc; 1981.

6. Brassard M, Ritter D. *The Memory Jogger II: A Pocket Guide of Tools for Continuous Improvement and Effective Planning.* Salem, NH: GOAL/QPC; 1994.

7. Walton M. *The Deming Management Method.* New York: Putnam Publishing; 1986.

8. Shewart WA. *The Economic Control of Quality of Manufactured Product.* New York: D. Van Nostrand Company; 1931. Reprinted by the American Society of Quality Control, 1980.

9. Lynn ML, Osborn DP. Deming's quality principles: a health care application. *Hosp Health Serv Adm.* 1991;6(1):111-20.

10. Deming WE. *Out of the Crisis.* Cambridge, MA: Massachusetts Institute of Technology; 1986.

11. Farris KB, Kirking DM. Assessing the quality of pharmaceutical care II. Application of concepts of quality assessment from medical care. *Ann Pharmacother.* 1993;27:215-23.

12. Donabedian A. Evaluating the quality of medical care. *Milbank Mem Fund Q.* 1966;44:166-203.

13. Donabedian A. The quality of care: how can it be assessed? *JAMA.* 1988;260(12):1743-48.

14. Farris KB, Kirking DM. Assessing the quality of pharmaceutical care I. One perspective of quality. *Ann Pharmacother.* 1993;27:68-73.

15. Kritchevsky SB, Simmons BP. Continuous quality improvement: concepts and applications for physician care. *JAMA.* 1991;266(13):1817-23.

16. Peters T. *Thriving on Chaos: Handbook for a Management Revolution.* New York: Alfred A. Knopf; 1991.

17. Langley GJ, Nolan KM, Nolan TW. The foundation of improvement. *Quality Progress.* 1994;27(6):81-6.

18. Moen RD, Nolan TW. Process improvement. *Quality Progress.* 1987;20(9):62-8.

19. Classen DC, Evans RS, Pestotnik SL, et al. The timing of prophylactic administration of antibiotics and the risk of surgical wound infection. *N Engl J Med.* 1992;326(5):281-86.

20. Cabana MD, Rand CS, Powe NR, et al. Why don't physicians follow clinical practice guidelines? *JAMA.* 1999;282(15):1458-65.

21. Ellrodt G, Cook DJ, Lee J, et al. Evidence-based disease management. *JAMA.* 1997;278(20):1687-92.

22. Deming WE. *Quality, Productivity, and Competitive Position.* Cambridge, MA: Massachusetts Institute of Technology Center for Advanced Engineering Study; 1982.

Index

Index

W
Ware, John, 186, 189
Washington State, pharmacy practice act
 of, 53
waste reduction, automation and, 79
wins, short-term, generating, 42–43
work activities
    in pharmacist job description, 128, 129
    in pharmacy operations, 81
    reassigning, 80–85
work activity analysis, 81–83
    calculating staffing adjustments with,
        83–84
    sample, 82t
work plan, 11–12, 12f. *See also* action plan
workflow, and pharmacy physical
 environment, 92

Y
Yurkovich, Nancy Jane, 25